LIVE LONGER
EAT BETTER

LIVE LONGER
EAT BETTER

Ancient Wisdom to Modern Tradition

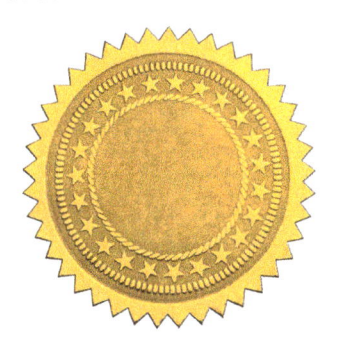

36 FOODS FOR LONG LIFE

Dr. E.A. Perry

MILL CITY PRESS

Mill City Press
555 Winderley Pl, Suite 225
Maitland, FL 32751
407.339.4217
www.millcitypress.net

© 2024 by Dr. E.A. Perry
Contributor: Professor Hsinpo Chen

All rights reserved solely by the author. The author guarantees all contents are original and do not infringe upon the legal rights of any other person or work. No part of this book may be reproduced in any form whatsoever without the permission of the author.

Due to the changing nature of the Internet, if there are any web addresses, links, or URLs included in this manuscript, these may have been altered and may no longer be accessible. The views and opinions shared in this book belong solely to the author and do not necessarily reflect those of the publisher. The publisher therefore disclaims responsibility for the views or opinions expressed within the work.

Paperback ISBN-13: 978-1-66289-191-5
Ebook ISBN-13: 978-1-66289-192-2

DEDICATION

I dedicate this book to Professor Hsinpo Chen, a distinguished Chinese scholar in the fields of Chinese culture and Traditional Chinese Medicine (TCM). Professor Chen has devoted many years researching this literature pertaining to ancient Chinese history of medicine, philosophy, and religions as well as how food therapy scientifically relates to TCM. He has taught food therapy at Atlantic Institute of Traditional Medicine for many years as well as Chinese language and culture at Florida International University (FIU) and Barry University. Without the teaching of Professor Chen, this book could not have been written.

PREFACE

The intention of this book is to help people live longer by eating better. I will share with you my own personal story and why I was inspired to write this book. Yes, I am a doctor, a Harvard graduate and a world traveler, but the root as to why I wrote this book and feel compelled to share food therapy is as follows:

One year and three months after I underwent a cesarean section for the birth of my child in 1989, I became extremely ill. I was seen and evaluated by some of the smartest and most highly trained doctors throughout the Boston area, ranging from expertise in primary care, endocrinology, obstetrics, infectious disease, nephrology, and psychiatry to name a few. I received textbook-perfect report cards by all, yet I was still so sick and weak. I was utterly exhausted and experienced intense chest oppression, cold sweats, severe chills, and violent seizure-like tremors, which were worse at night, yet to touch my body was to feel it burning up. I had a fever of over 100 degrees for a year and a half, and I was only twenty-three years old. I was bedbound and had to have help with basic daily activities.

No doctor that I'd seen was able to identify, diagnose, or treat my condition. It was simply awful. The World Wide Web had not yet been launched, so I had been contributing my time to the local library prior to the onset of this illness and had a relationship with the staff. I decided to call the chief librarian to ask if she would research journals and publications for celebrities having such symptoms. She found two, Cherilyn Sarkisian (otherwise known as Cher) and Chrystie Brinkley. According to these articles, they had both been diagnosed with what some referred to as Chronic Fatigue Syndrome (CFS). Cher's story was compelling. Why? Because she had been largely debilitated, like myself, and her story offered a solution. According to the article, she improved her condition by using food therapy alongside other remedies such as herbal, visualization, and Tai Chi exercises. I decided to emulate the protocols she had used. Chrystie Brinkley also used food therapy to heal. Due to the glory of God, the help of the librarian, and strategic food therapy along with Tai Chi and visualization exercises, my condition began to improve. I started to recognize the power of food.

There is no argument that the invention of antibiotics is a miracle and innovative technologies for surgical intervention indubitably helps save lives. In my case, however, along with millions of others, food therapy was effective in resolving my health condition, whereas surgery or antibiotics were not.

I met an interesting predecessor, a *Harvard alum,* from the business school while I was in my first year at Harvard. We spoke about various verticals, healthcare leadership, Abu, Dubai, and Harvard education. He encouraged world travel for a year following graduation. He implied that by doing such, it would become clear as to what the world really needed. He was a wise visionary and he was right. I traveled the world and realized what was needed, a healthier health system in America. Other countries did better at preventing disease, treating viruses, and treating chronic conditions. Why is that? After all, America is supposed to be the best!

Upon my return, I attended medical school where I studied biomedicine, Chinese medicine, German medicine, and strategic protocols used in Russia. Food therapy was used with each patient and as part of the total treatment plan in nearly every condition.

Traditional Chinese Medicine (TCM) theory is one of the oldest medical systems and has a profound understanding of humanity, health systems, universal systems, and the perfect square, *Tao Te Ching*. The most brilliant, highly evolved mathematicians, NASA physicists, and scholars know this, too, and only wish they had many more lifetimes to further study the perfect square and how it holds solution to all problems.

TCM's unique and brilliant knowledge of pathophysiology through meridian organ systems bring such powerful significance to the medical field.

With over thirty years in the healthcare field, globally, it is clear that Americans benefit by using biomedicine, but could benefit further by incorporating other effective practices from around the world, such as TCM. This ancient theory and practice can effectively treat not only trauma and acute health problems, but bacterial, fungal, and viral infections and numerous chronic diseases. So, it just makes sense to have more doctors of acupuncture and oriental medicine experts trained and available here in the United States. The wise ancient medical literature states:

> Superior practitioners treat diseases before they arise and get 90 percent cure rate. Mediocre practitioner treats what is ill already and gets 70 percent cure rate. Inferior doctors treat the full-blown disease and often have less than a 60 percent success rate.

To become a superior practitioner, food therapy is of significant importance to the winning formula of preventative strategy and long-life plan for human life.

I credit Michael Greger, MD, FACLM for taking a key leadership role in educating the American public on the importance of food and its impact while backing it by science (https://www.nutritionfacts.org). He is absolutely brilliant, highly influential, and considered one of the greatest assets to the American Healthcare System in over a century.

As the author of this book, I simply attempt to consolidate knowledge of food, from the old and the new, to help patients know what to eat and why, using wisdom of the Tao and modern research and meta-analysis, which follows much of the work that Dr. Michael Greger has compiled.

Sadly, so many patients come in to my office, be it COVID or cancer, asking, "What should we be eating?" Patients are being told by conventional medical practitioners that food is not relevant to their disease. That, my friends, is simply a false statement.

It matters. Food matters. There is science behind food. Food has a powerful and proven influence on our well-being. It may not be the total solution in each and every case, but it is an effective modality and must be respected and utilized in each and every medical solution. I will say this again: food matters! I know this as a patient, as a data analyst, as a researcher, and as a doctor of acupuncture and oriental medicine.

TABLE OF CONTENTS

Section I 36 FOODS FOR LONG LIFE 1

1. ASPARAGUS 2
2. BAMBOO SHOOTS 3
3. BANANA 4
4. BIE JIA / SOFSHELL TURTLE 5
5. BLACK BEANS 6
6. BLACK/WHITE FUNGUS / WOOD EAR MUSHROOMS 7
7. CELERY 8
8. CHESTNUTS 9
9. CHINES YAM / SWEET POTATO 10
10. CORN 11
11. CUCUMBER 12
12. DATES (RED) / JUJUBE 13
13. EGGPLANT 14
14. FISH, CHICKEN, DUCK, AND MEATS 15
15. GARLIC 16
16. GINGER 17
17. GRAPES 18
18. HONEY 19
19. KELP (HAI DAI) 20
20. LOTUS SEEDS 21
21. MILK 22
22. MUSHROOMS 23
23. ONIONS 24
24. PEANUTS 25
25. POTATO 26
26. RABBIT 27
27. RADISH 28
28. RICE 29
29. ROYAL JELLY 30
30. SESAME SEEDS 31
31. SHAN ZHA / HAWTHORN 32
32. SOYBEANS 33
33. SPINACH 34
34. TOMATOS 35
35. WALNUTS 36
36. WATERMELON 37

Section II WORLD OF WISDOM (W.O.W.) QUIZ 39

Section III ASK DR. LIZ 63

1. ACUPUNCTURE 65
2. ALCOHOL 67
3. LET'S PREVENT ALZEIMER'S 69
4. AN APPLE A DAY 71
5. AVACADO 72
6. GOING BANANAS? 73
7. ALZHEIMER'S AND CANDIDA 74
8. CELERY 75
9. ARE YOU CHICKEN? 76
10. BENEFITS OF COCONUT OIL 77
11. TELL ME ABOUT DEPRESSION 78
12. DIABETES 82
13. ENERGY DENSITY 83
14. FERTILITY: TIPS FOR GETTING PREGNANT 84
15. FOLK REMEDY VS. TCM 85
16. GUT HEALTH 87
17. HEART HEALTH AND CARDIOVASCULAR DISEASE 88
18. FOODS FOR HEART HEALTH 93
19. HI, HONEY! 94
20. KIDNEY DISEASE 96
21. DIET FOR KIDNEY HEALTH 98
22. MUSHROOMS 100
23. NUTRITIONAL YEAST 101
24. LET'S GO NUTS! 102
25. OXIDATIVE STRESS 103
26. HOW MUCH PROTEIN IS IDEAL AS WE AGE? 104
27. PRUNES FOR OSTEOPEROSIS! 105
28. SEAWEED 106
29. SESAME SEEDS 107
30. FOODS FOR BETTER SEX 109
31. QUIT SMOKING 110
32. TEA TIME 111
33. VITAMIN D: THE "SUNSHINE" VITAMIN 112
34. WATERMELON 113
35. WEIGHT LOSS AND DIABETES 115
36. FOODS FOR LONG LIFE 117

INTRODUCTION

The primary focus of this book, *Live Longer–Eat Better* is to bridge the gap between ancient wisdom and modern tradition when it comes to food therapy. This book has three sections and is designed to be used as a general guide.

Section I, "36 Foods for Long Life," is based on the great wisdom of the Tao.

Section II, the "World of Wisdom (W.O.W.) Quiz," helps to identify your personal constitution and which organ pathway needs attention. Foods are suggested based on your results of the quiz.

Section III, "Ask Dr Liz," are thirty-six short, yet informative articles on food that are based on meta-analysis and clinical research.

Acupuncturists, doctors of oriental medicine, and TCM scholars are knowledgeable about which organ system food actually goes to and what the function of the food is. In Section I, I introduce you to a new way to look at food, a mini knowledge base of what a doctor of acupuncture and oriental medicine can further provide you with. Exercising this awareness alongside modern nutritional value and clinical studies can help you become more vital and alive. This is likely new information to most people from the West. I do my best to provide you this complex knowledge in the simplest way.

For example, alcohol goes to the heart first, not the liver, which is why people who consume too much often have a full red face. In TCM, we know that a full red face shows there is heat in the heart or the heart organ pathway; therefore, it is indicative of a heart pathology. Similarly, in modern science, there is a very clear link between consuming too much alcohol and high blood pressure. People with hypertension commonly present with a full red face. The wisdom of the Tao and knowledge of modern medicine, where East meets West, conclude similarly. The distinction is modern science attempts to explain food therapy in terms of vitamins, minerals, and phytonutrients whereas TCM explains specific properties of each food, which organ system it goes to, and what the primary function of the food is.

Another example is the carrot. Many of us were told by our parents as children that carrots will improve your vision and the health of your eyes. Our parents were right. Modern science attempts to justify this wisdom using clinical research studies of carotenoids, beta-carotene, and phytochemicals, and they do so successfully. Ancient wisdom of the Tao or TCM knows the carrot goes to the liver, lungs, and spleen organ system within the body. The liver meridian, or organ pathway, controls the health of the eyes. The carrot not only goes to the eyes by entering the liver channel organ system, but the function of the carrot is to create circulation behind the eyes. Modern science arrives at the similar knowledge and outcome, but the ancients have known this strategically and scientifically for thousands of years.

In Section I, you will notice these abbreviations seen below. This will allow you to see which organ pathway each of the thirty-six foods for long life goes to":

See the chart below to identify organ system and meridian pathway abbreviations:

GB = Gallbladder	HT = Heart	KD = Kidney	LI = Large Intestine
LV = Liver	LU = Lung	SI = Small Intestine	SP = Spleen
ST = Stomach	UB = Bladder		

More from the Tao

Healthy food consumption is necessary for long life. Taoism explores how to live a quality, and graceful long life consuming foods that are natural, seasonal and fresh. Diets and food intake are a highly personal experience. Both Ayurvedic Medicine and TCM originate from the great wisdom of the Tao, and effectively use food therapy as a modality to prevent and treat disease.

Other consideration must be taken into account to optimize our vitality and lifespan when it comes to food, including preparation and timing of the food you eat, seasonal food choices, temperature of food and drink, and climate changes. Changing our diet as we age and our constitution changes is also key in optimizing our bodies as we evolve.

If you want to live longer, what can you do to make this happen? Common threads that lead to longevity in addition to food therapy include activities such as spending time with nature, meditating, maintaining a positive mental attitude, staying involved, and moving often. People who live the longest often care about something outside of themselves.

In Section II, you are invited to take the W.O.W. Quiz, where you will be asked a series of quick questions. Don't overthink them. Just answer yes or no as to whether each question pertains to you or not. By doing so, you will get clarity as to which organ system needs attention. For example, if you have constant night sweats, a dry mouth, and low back pain, you will benefit from eating foods that nourish the kidney organ system.

In Section III, articles are based predominantly on modern science and contemporary clinical research. These articles are designed to be informative in preventing disease through the use of food.

The objective of this book is to perhaps inspire a new awareness to food therapy, it's importance to prevention and healing, and the added brilliance and great wisdom of the Tao. By combining wisdom from the Tao with modern science and nutrition, you gain a World of Wisdom (W.O.W.) and can optimally prepare you for a long, vital life.

SECTION 1

36 FOODS FOR LONG LIFE

1. ASPARAGUS
2. BAMBOO SHOOTS
3. BANANA
4. BIE JIA/ SOFTSHELL TURTLE
5. BLACK BEANS
6. BLACK/WHITE FUNGUS / WOOD EAR MUSHROOMS
7. CELERY
8. CHESTNUTS
9. CHINESE YAM / SWEET POTATO
10. CORN
11. CUCUMBER
12. DATES (RED) / JUJUBE
13. EGGPLANT
14. FISH, CHICKEN, DUCK, AND MEATS
15. GARLIC
16. GINGER
17. GRAPES
18. HONEY
19. KELP (HAI DAI)
20. LOTUS SEEDS
21. MILK
22. MUSHROOMS
23. ONIONS
24. PEANUTS
25. POTATO
26. RABBIT
27. RADISH
28. RICE
29. ROYAL JELLY
30. SESAME SEEDS
31. SHAN ZHA / HAWTHORN
32. SOYBEANS
33. SPINACH
34. TOMATO
35. WALNUTS
36. WATERMELON

#1–ASPARAGUS
ANTI-CANCER FOOD

Ancient Wisdom: Top ten vegetable of the world.

Flavor: Sweet, slightly bitter
Temperature: Cool, cold
Function:
    Anti-aging
    Builds the blood
    Calms the liver
    Clears heat
    Reduces edema
    Treats constipation, cough, diabetes, and hemoptysis

Organ System: KD, LU, LV, SP

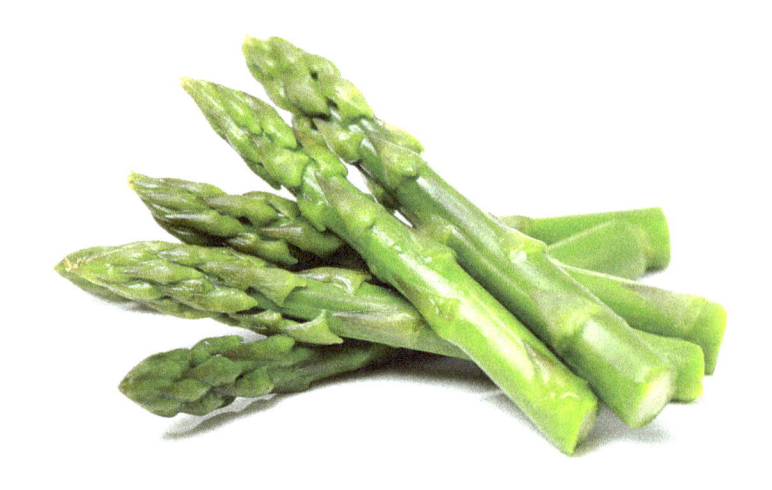

Modern Tradition

Helps prevent and treat cancer, including but not limited to adenocarcinoma, breast, colon, endometrial, pancreatic, and prostate. Contains a rich source of antioxidants, minerals, saponins, and vitamins. Saponins boost immunity, improve RBC anemia, lowers blood pressure, promotes healthy pregnancy, promotes weight loss, reduces stress, stabilizes blood sugar, and treats constipation.

#2–BAMBOO SHOOTS
ANTI-CANCER FOOD

Ancient Wisdom: Bamboo shoots have lots of protein and vitamins contained within.

Flavor: Sweet
Temperature: Cold
Function:
    Fights against cardiovascular disease
    Helps to prevent and treats cancer
    Improves immunity powerfully
    Lubricates large intestine channel and treats constipation
    Reduces renal reperfusion, a condition linked to kidney failure
    Transforms phlegm with heat
    Anti-bacterial, anti-cancer, and anti-viral

Organ System: GB, LI, LU, ST

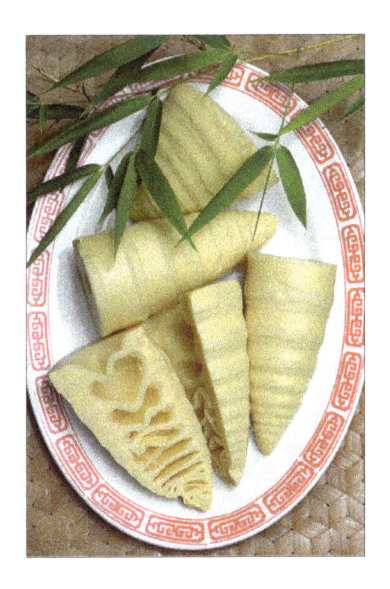

Modern Tradition

Nutrient rich containing amino acids, fiber, minerals, phytosterols, and vitamins including calcium, copper, magnesium, manganese, potassium, phosphorus, thiamin (B1), riboflavin (B2), niacin (B3), pyridoxine (B6), vitamin A, and vitamin E. Good for adrenals and thyroid glands, digestion, and hair growth. Improves appetite, lowers cholesterol, regulates blood sugar, and regulates hormones. Treats ADHD.

#3–BANANA

Ancient Wisdom: Number one fruit with world athletes

Flavor: Sweet
Temperature: Cold
Function:
    Aids in digestion
    Boosts mood
    Clears heat in the large intestine channel
    Enhances heart health
    Improves blood pressure and stomach ulcers
    Stops bleeding hemorrhoids
    Treats constipation and high cholesterol
    Quenches thirst
Organ System: KD, LI, LV

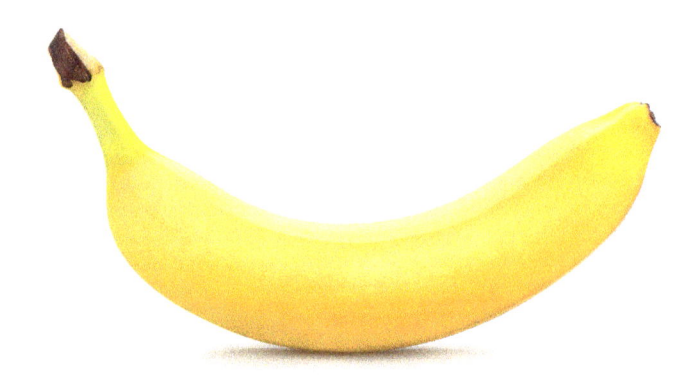

Modern Tradition

Provides instant, sustainable energy boost. High in potassium, low in salt. Reduces the risk of hypertension and stroke, according to the FDA. Reduces stress and depression. Promotes weight loss and treats constipation.

#4–BIE JIA / SOFTSHELL TURTLE
ANTI-CANCER FOOD

Ancient Wisdom:

Flavor: Salty
Temperature: Cool, slightly cold
Function:
- A great yin tonic
- Anchors the yang
- Boosts immunity
- Calms the shen
- Clears heat and eliminates night sweats
- Improves blood circulation
- Tonifies the heart and kidney
- Treats hot flashes and menopausal symptoms
- Anti-aging, anti-cancer

Organ System: KD, HT, LV

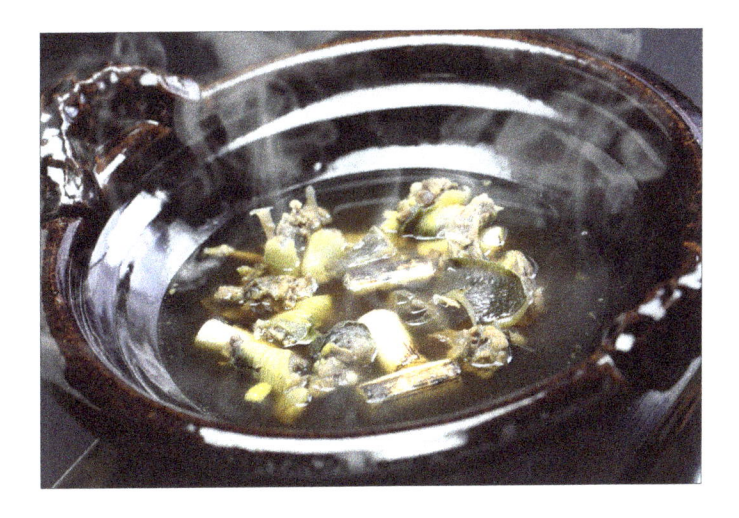

Modern Tradition

Has little fat and contains rich nutrients including iron, potassium, selenium, vitamin B1 (thiamin), vitamin B2 (riboflavin), vitamin B12, and zinc. Treats anemia, fever, malaria, rickets, and seizures. Enhances amelioration of bone mesenchymal stem cells on hepatocellular carcinoma progression.

#5–BLACK BEANS

Ancient Wisdom: Grains of the kidney.

Flavor: Sweet
Temperature: Cool, neutral
Function:
- Protect the kidneys
- Detoxify the liver and are highly nutritious
- Help to prevent and treat constipation
- Promotes healthy bacteria in colon
- Promotes regularity
- Treats low back pain and knee pain
- Strengthens digestion and brightens the eyes
- Treats aspects of infertility and seminal emissions

Organ System: KD, LV, SP

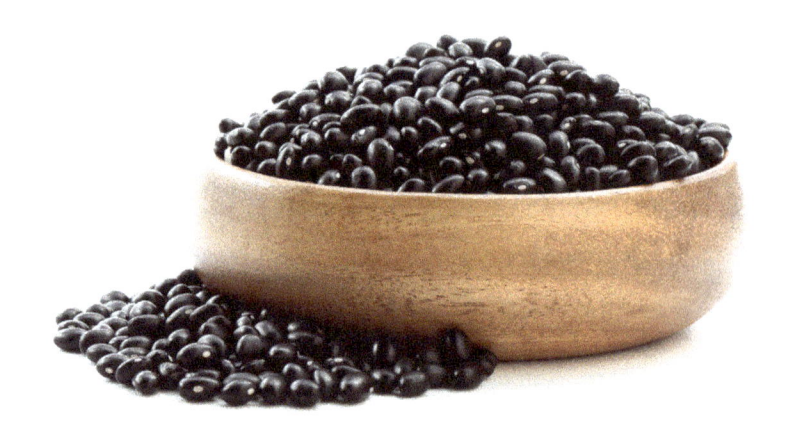

Modern Tradition

Regulates blood pressure, blood sugar, cholesterol, and improves cardiovascular health and gut health. Protects against cancer and neurodegenerative disease. Promotes mineral absorption.

#6 – BLACK/WHITE FUNGUS / WOOD EAR MUSHROOMS

Ancient Wisdom:

Flavor: Sweet
Temperature: Neutral
Black Fungus Function:
    Cools blood
    Moistens dryness
    Stops excess vaginal bleeding (especially effective in post child birth bleeding)
    Stops hemorrhoid bleeding
    Tonifies the stomach
    Treats sharp shooting pain
    White Fungus Function:
    Can moisten the lungs
    Nourish the yin
    Promote saliva
    Tonify the brain and the heart
Organ System: LV, LU, ST

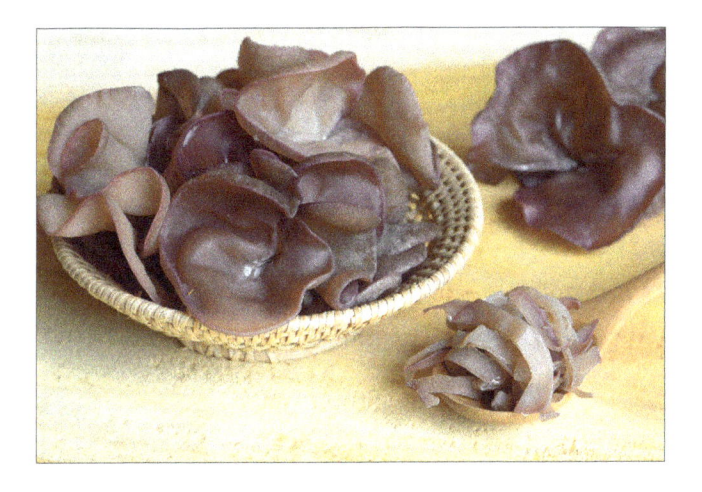

Modern Tradition

Rich in antioxidants and fiber. Aids in weight loss, anti-inflammatory, improves circulation, lowers cholesterol, promotes gut health, and protects liver.

#7–CELERY

Ancient Wisdom: Good for people with arteriosclerosis, hypertension, and poor nerves.

Flavor: Bitter, sweet
Temperature: Cool
Function:
    Clears damp heat
    Dispels wind
    Good for arteriosclerosis and nervous system
    Improves urinary problems
    Treats abscesses, diarrhea, and dysentery
    Lowers high blood pressure
    Strengthens the stomach
    Tranquilizes the mind
    Treats red eyes, swelling, and vertigo

Organ System: LV, ST

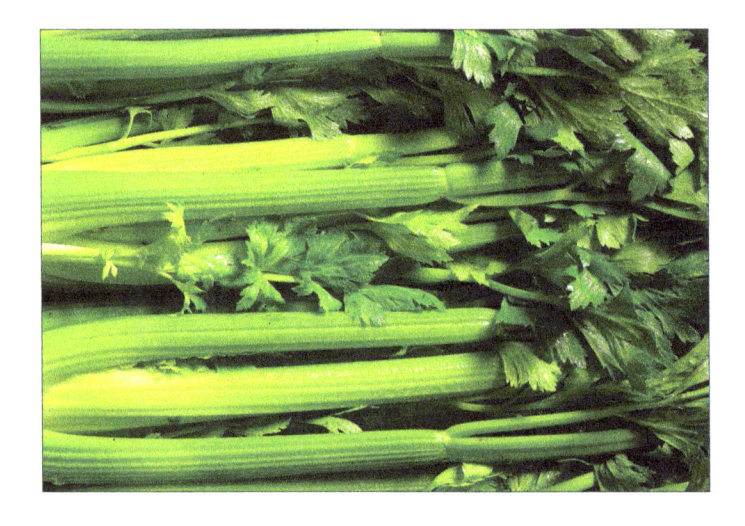

Modern Tradition

Anti-bacterial, anti-inflammatory, and anti-viral. Aids in weight loss. Diuretic, good for heart health, improves memory, regulates blood sugar. Contains luteolin, is good for the brain, and prevents inflammation in the brain cells. Relaxes artery walls and lowers blood pressure. Contains DL-3-n-butylphthalide, improves learning, thinking and memory. Research suggests that celery strengthens the heart and reduces arterial plaque.

#8–CHESTNUTS

Ancient Wisdom: King of the preserved fruits.

Flavor: Sweet
Temperature: Warm
Function:
    Enlivens the blood
    Especially good for people with kidney deficiency
    Improves the condition of the ligaments and tendons
    Stops nose bleeds
    Strengthens the kidneys
    Treats arteriosclerosis, bruises, coronary disease, hypertension, and lower back pain

Organ System: KD, SP, ST

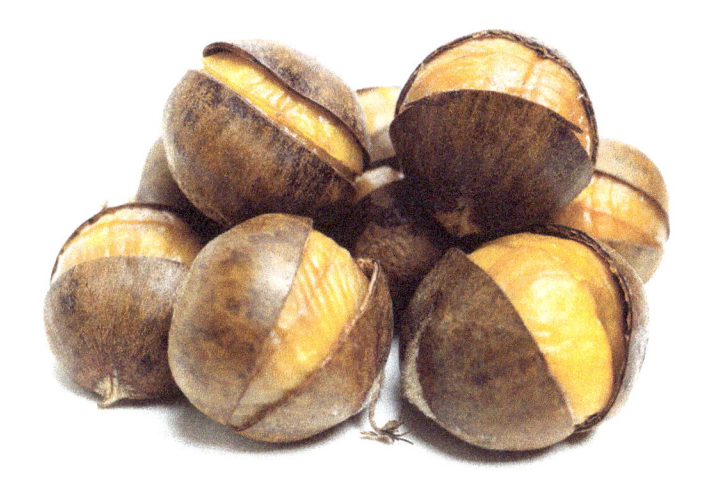

Modern Tradition

High in antioxidants and phytosterols, arginine, selenium, vitamin C, and collagen. Research suggests reduction of abdominal adipose and regulates adipose tissue deposition. Good for joints and arthritic conditions.

#9–CHINESE YAM / SWEET POTATO
ANTI-AGING FOOD

Ancient Wisdom:

Flavor: Sweet
Chinese Yam Temperature: Neutral, warm,
Sweet Potato Temperature: Cool
Chinese Yam Function:
    Tonifies the middle jiao, kidneys, and lungs.
    Improves digestion
    Anti-aging food
    Sweet Potato Function:
    Boosts energy
    Good for diabetes
    Improves digestion
    Regulates bowels
    Treats constipation, diarrhea, fatigue, and premature ejaculation
    Chinese Yam Organ System: KD, LU, SP
Sweet Potato Organ System: SP, ST

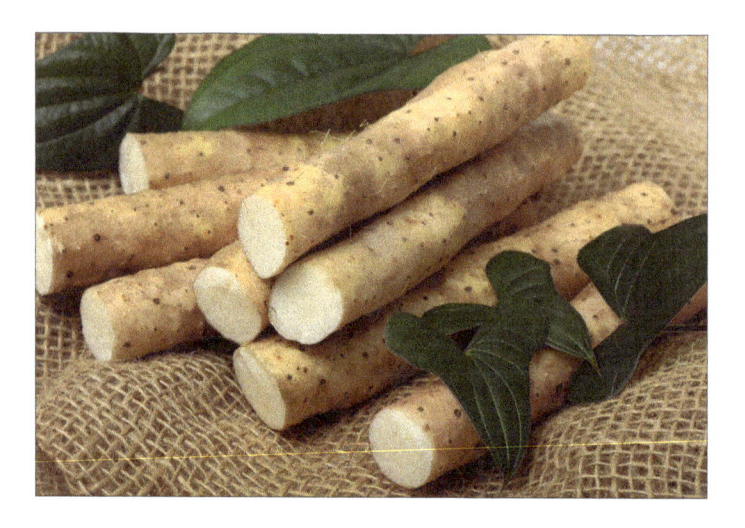

Modern Tradition

High in vitamin B, vitamins C, and fiber. Improves eye health, gut health, immunity, and is good for the brain. Helps regulate hormone production for women by stimulating production of progesterone.

#10–CORN
ANTI-CANCER FOOD

Ancient Wisdom: The golden grain.

Flavor: Sweet
Temperature: Neutral
Function:
    Protects the heart and blood vessels
    Reduces cholesterol
    Treats gallstones, difficult urination, hepatitis, hypertension, and jaundice
Organ System: BL, GB, HT, LV, LU, SP, ST

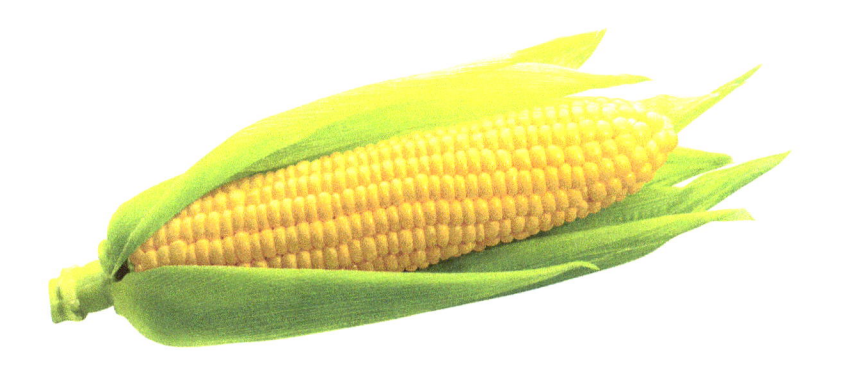

Modern Tradition

Aids in digestion, improves vision, and protects the heart. Yellow sweet corn is an excellent source of lutein and zeaxanthin. It is an anti-inflammatory containing phenolic acids and flavonoids.

#11–CUCUMBER
ANTI-CANCER FOOD

Ancient Wisdom:

Flavor: Sweet
Temperature: Cool, cold
Function:
> Has anti-cancer elements due to the beta-carotene contained
> Improves urinary problems
> Reduces fever and swelling
> Treats cough

Organ System: BL, LI, SP, ST

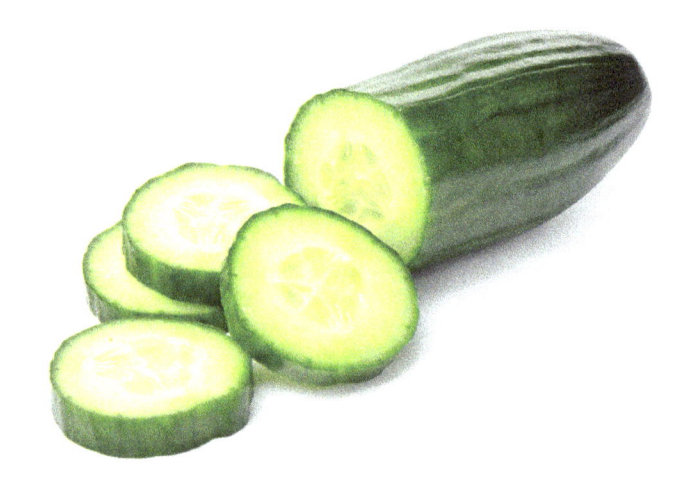

Modern Tradition

Cucumbers are natural detoxifiers and anti-inflammatories. They increase hydration, are high in vitamin K and potassium, strengthen bones, promote gut health, help stabilize blood sugar, promote weight loss, improves heart health, and is an anti-cancer food.

#12–DATES (RED) / JUJUBE

Ancient Wisdom: A woman looks just like a teenager at the age of fifty just because she ate dates as a staple food.

Flavor: Sweet
Temperature: Warm
Function:
    Benefits the qi
    Boosts energy level
    Harmonizes the stomach
    Rich in vitamin
    Tonifies the spleen
    Treats fatigue, hysteria, and shortness of breath

*According to the book *Bei Meng Suo Yan*, a British scientist thinks of dates as the natural vitamin supplier.

Organ System: SP, ST

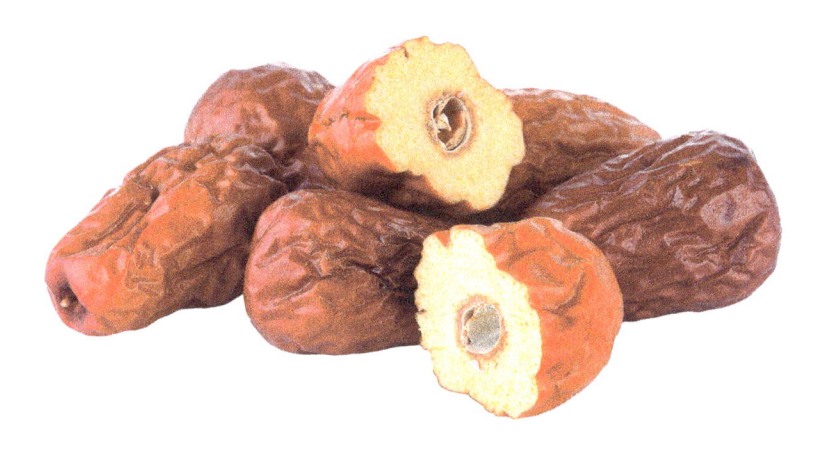

Modern Tradition

Aids digestion, alleviates stress, and expectorant. Improves brain health, immunity, loose stools, loss of appetite, memory, and sleep. Good for weight loss. Lowers cholesterol and risk of colorectal cancer. Treats ADHD. Antiallergic, antimutagenic, antineoplastic, antioxidant, and antitussive.

#13–EGGPLANT

Ancient Wisdom: Number one vegetable different from all other vegetables.

Flavor: Sweet
Temperature: Cool
Function:
    Contains more vitamin PP than any other fruit or vegetable
    An excellent protection against most cardiovascular diseases by protecting blood vessels
    Treats bleeding hemorrhoids and sellings
Organ System: LI, ST, SP

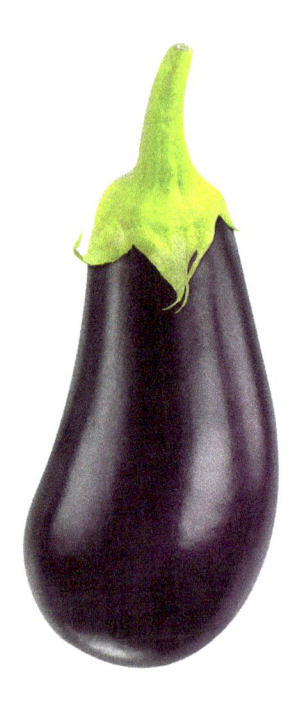

Modern Tradition

Promotes weight loss, reduces risk of heart disease, and stabilizes blood sugar. Anti-cancer food.

#14–FISH, CHICKEN, DUCK, AND MEATS

Ancient Wisdom: Ninety-six percent of a fish's nutrients can be absorbed.

Flavor: Fish (White): Sweet / Chicken: Sweet / Duck: Sweet and salty / Beef: Sweet / Pork: Sweet and salty
Temperature: Fish: Neutral / Chicken: Warm / Duck: Neutral / Beef: Warm / Pork: Neutral
Fish (White) Function: Includes bass, catfish, cod, flounder, grouper, haddock, snapper, and tilapia
Chicken Function: Circulates blood and disperses cold, and tonifies Qi, blood, and jing
Duck: Builds blood, resolves dampness, regulates water, and tonifies QI, blood, and yin
Beef: Number one food for RBC anemia, builds blood, helps boosts yang, tonifies QI, blood, and yin, and warms the body
Pork: Tonifies QI, blood, and yin

Organ System: Fish: LU, LV, SP, ST / Chicken: KD, SP, ST / Duck: KD, LU, SP, ST / Beef: LI, LV, SP, ST / Pork: KD, LV, SP, ST

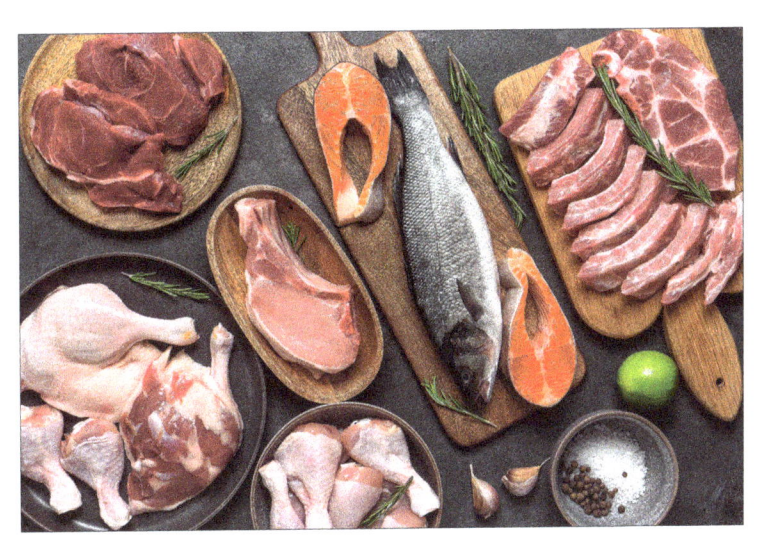

Modern Tradition

Fish is loaded with nutrients, proteins, and vitamins than can lower blood pressure and reduces risk of heart attack and stroke.
Chicken can improve brain function, build muscle, strengthen bones, and aid in weight loss. Contains (B6) thiamin, pantothenic acid, copper, iron, and zinc.
Duck (White Pekin) contains vitamins A, B1, B2, and K, increases energy levels, and helps increase good cholesterol levels.
Pork contains B6, B12, iron, and selenium. It is good for brain function and thyroid health.
Beef is the best source of iron rich food to treat RBC anemia.

#15–GARLIC
ANTI-CANCER FOOD

Ancient Wisdom: Helps prevent Alzheimer's disease and dementia.

Flavor: Acrid
Temperature: Warm
Function:
- Anti-aging drug, anti-bacteria, antibiotic, and anti-cancer
- Protects blood vessels
- Treats bloating, diarrhea, malaria, whooping cough, and abscesses
- Reduces blood stasis

Organ System: SP, ST, LU

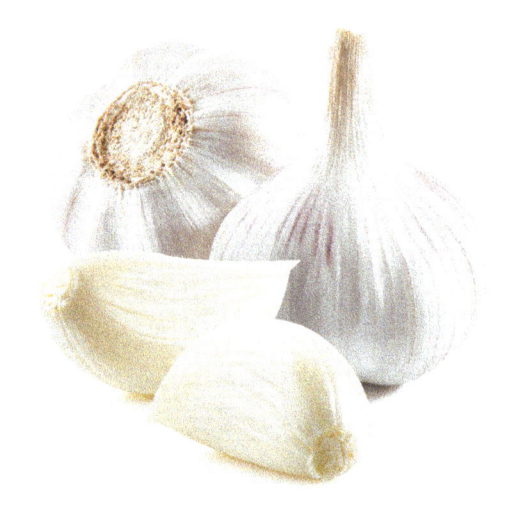

Modern Tradition

Anti-cancer food, boosts immunity, lowers blood pressure, expedites wound healing. It is a natural antibiotic and can significantly reduce risk of atherosclerosis, cholesterol, diabetes, hypertension, and can reduce ALT and AST liver enzymes. Promotes weight loss.

#16–GINGER
ANTI-CANCER FOOD

Ancient Wisdom:

Flavor: Acrid
Temperature: Slightly warm
Function:
    Stops nausea and vomiting
    Transforms phlegm
    Treats cold, flu, and cough
    Disperses the wind and cold
    Lowers blood pressure and blood fat
    Refrains the growth of cancer cells

Organ System: LU, SP, ST

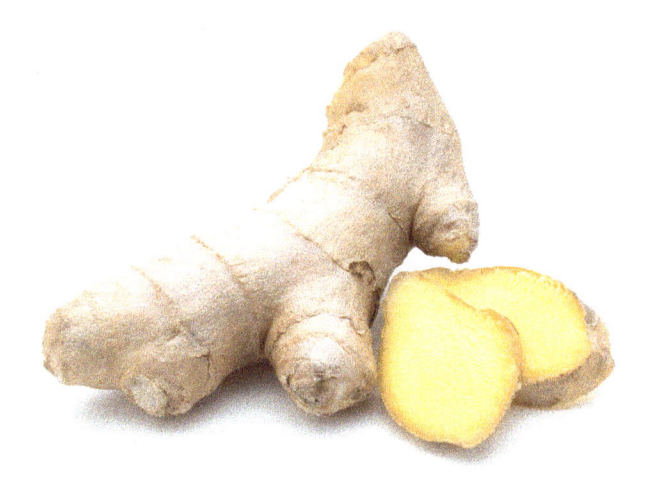

Modern Tradition

Ginger boosts brain function, lowers cholesterol, fights infections, treats nausea and stomach pain, helps digestion, bloating and gas. Anti-bacterial. Good for weight loss.

#17-GRAPES

Ancient Wisdom: Promotes brain health and improves memory.

Flavor: Sweet, sour
Temperature: Neutral
Function:
    A diuretic
    Strengthens ligaments, tendons, and bones
    Treats edema, night sweats, and heart palpitations
    Disinhibits urine
    Good for qi and blood
    Helps with weak stomach and spleen
    Does away with wind and dampness
    Tonifies all sorts of deficiency

Organ System: KD, LU, SP

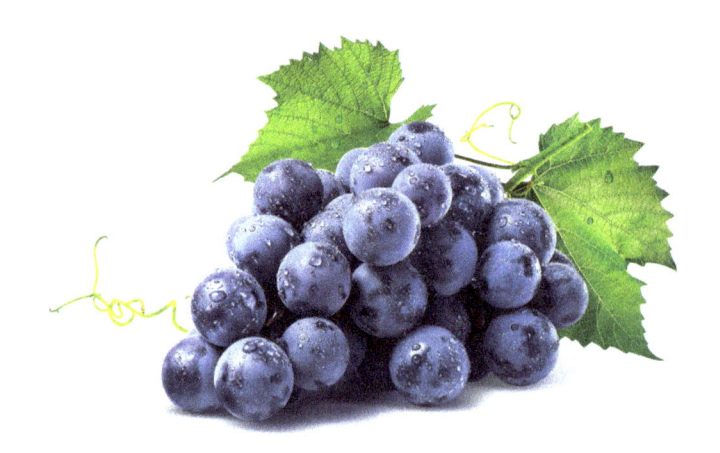

Modern Tradition

Anti-aging. Boosts immunity, improves eye health, hydration, heart health, promotes sleep, protects eyes, and protects against insulin resistance. Good for bone health.

#18–HONEY

Ancient Wisdom: A friend of good health.

Flavor: Sweet
Temperature: Neutral
Function:
    Externally treats mouth sores and scalding burns
    Has effects of killing bacteria
    Moistens the intestines
    Treats cough and constipation
    Protects the liver
    Good protector against cancers of the nose and throat

Organ System: LU, SP, LI

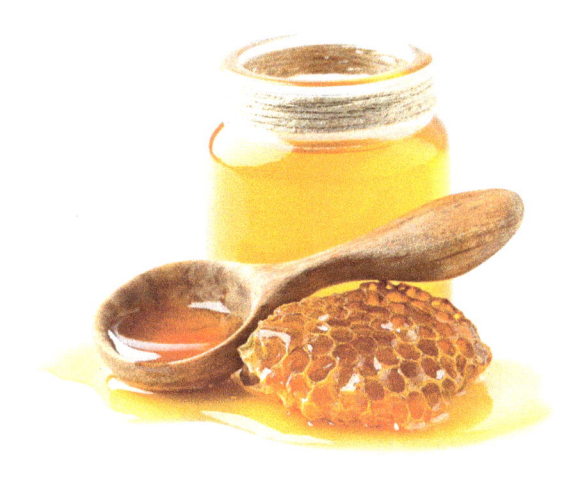

Modern Tradition

Anti-depressant, anti-convulsant, anti-anxiety, improves wound healing, and improves memory.

#19 – KELP (HAI DAI)

Ancient Wisdom:

Flavor: Salty
Temperature: Cold
Function:
    Disinhibits water
    Drains heat
    Softens hardness
    Transforms phlegm and helps treat foot problems ranging from athlete's foot to pain
    Treats swellings
    Rich in vitamin A and B2
    Reduces blood stasis and chronic inflammation
    Very rich in iodine
    Treats night blindness and thyroid gland enlargement
Organ System: KD, LV, LU, ST

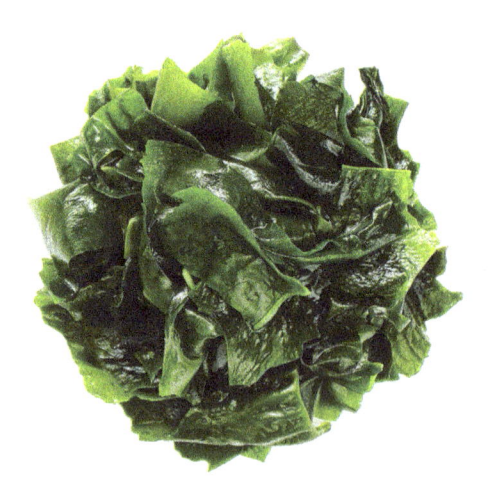

Modern Tradition

Anti-aging, anti-inflammatory, boosts energy levels and metabolism. Improves type 2 diabetes, strengthens bones, treats gastric ulcers, improves thyroid function, promotes weight loss, and reduces hair loss.

#20–LOTUS SEEDS
ANTI-CANCER FOOD

Ancient Wisdom:

Flavor: Sweet, astringent
Temperature: Neutral
Function:
>Anti-aging
>Helps to prevent and treat cancer of the nose and throat
>Treats diarrhea, insomnia, palpitations, poor appetite, premature ejaculation, and restlessness

*Listed as a superb food in *Shennong Bencaojing*. Lotus seeds can live for thousands of years. Ben Cao Bei Yao wrote, "When they fall down in the field, we pick them up to eat them and will remain young with a good head of black hair."

Organ System: HT, KD, SP

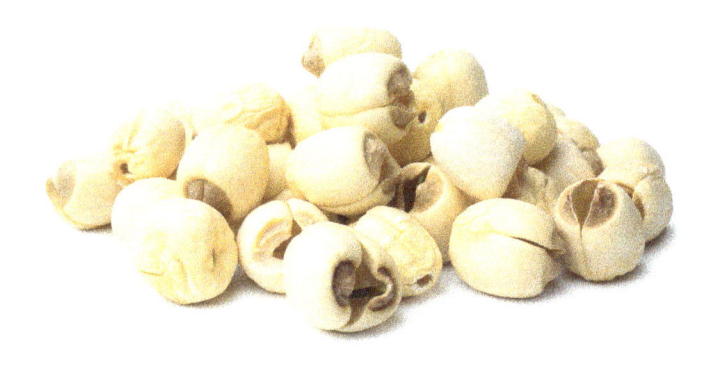

Modern Tradition

Aids weight loss, anti-inflammatory. Enhances kidney health, low glycemic index, promotes heart health, stabilizes blood sugar, and treats insomnia and palpitations.

#21–MILK
COMPREHENSIVE NUTRIENTS

Ancient Wisdom:

Flavor: Sweet
Temperature: Neutral
Function:
    Helps diabetes
    Treats constipation
Organ System: HT, LU, ST

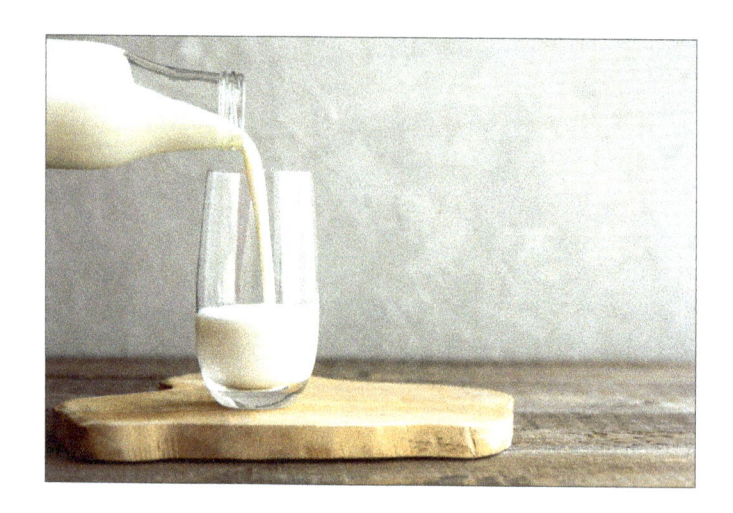

Modern Tradition

Aids digestion, balances mood, boosts immunity, improves hair and skin, and strengthens bones and teeth.

#22–MUSHROOMS
ANTI-CANCER FOOD

Ancient Wisdom: Treats fatigue.

Flavor: Sweet
Temperature: Cool
Function:
    Quiets the Spirit
    Resolves Rashes
    Transforms Phlegm

*1 kilo of mushrooms equals 2 kilos of lean meat, 3 kilos of chicken eggs, and 12 kilos of milk in terms of protein.

*Mushrooms can regulate the qi circulation, increase immunity. White fungus can promote the saliva, moisten the lungs, nourish the yin, and tonify the brain and heart. Anti-cancer function.

*Black mushrooms contain sixteen kinds of amino acids. They can strengthen the stomach and benefit the qi, increase immunity, treat anemia, hypertension, high blood sugar, reduce fat, treat diabetes, and arteriosclerosis.

Organ System: LI, LU, ST

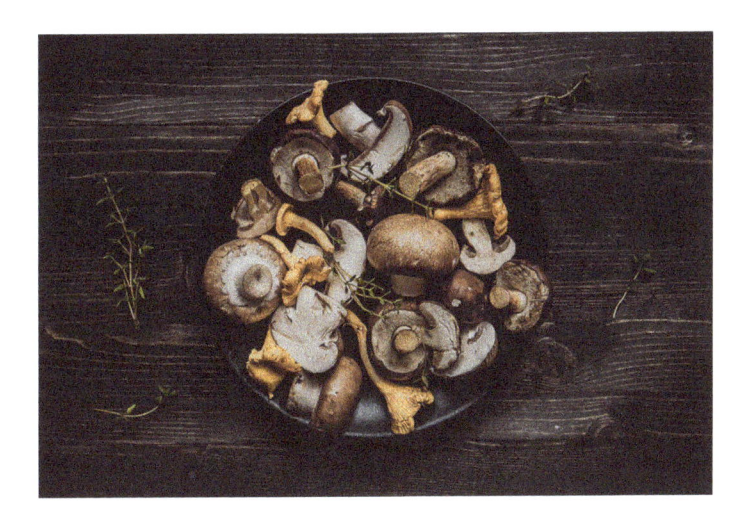

Modern Tradition

Shitake mushrooms, also known as black fungus and the scientific name is lentinus edo, are high in B and D vitamins, aid in weight loss, improve cardiovascular health, fight cancer cells, and improve energy levels, brain function, and immune function. Reduces inflammation, lowers cholesterol, and improves gut health.

#23–ONION
ANTI-CANCER FOOD

Ancient Wisdom:

Flavor: Acrid
Temperature: Warm
Function:
    Treats cold, flu, diarrhea, and worms
    Can expand the blood vessels, lower blood pressure, and blood fat
    A diuretic
Organ System: LI ,LU, LV, SP

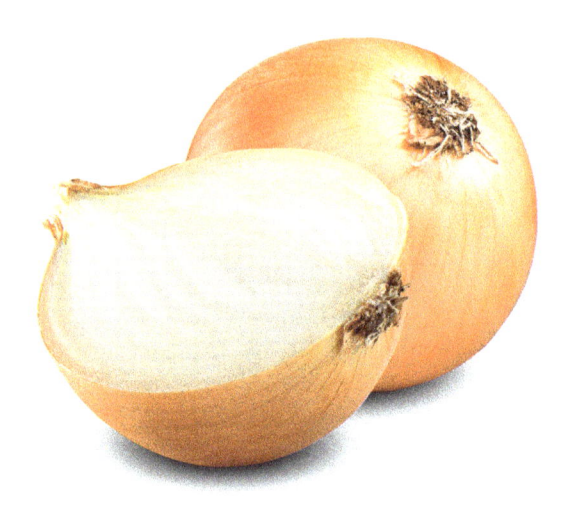

Modern Tradition

Stabilize blood sugar, improves digestion, anti-inflammatory, high level of vitamin C, and reduces risk of Alzheimer's disease.

#24–PEANUTS

Ancient Wisdom: Longevity nut, botanical meat.

Flavor: Sweet
Temperature: Neutral
Function:
    Contains 50 percent oil, twice as much as soy beans
    Good for the brain
    Harmonies the stomach
    Has rich, unsaturated fatty acid, vitamin E, and more than twenty kinds of chemicals and vitamins
    Good for the brain
    Moistens the lungs
    Stops bleeding
    Treats dry cough, nausea, and scanty lactation
Organ System: LU, SP, ST

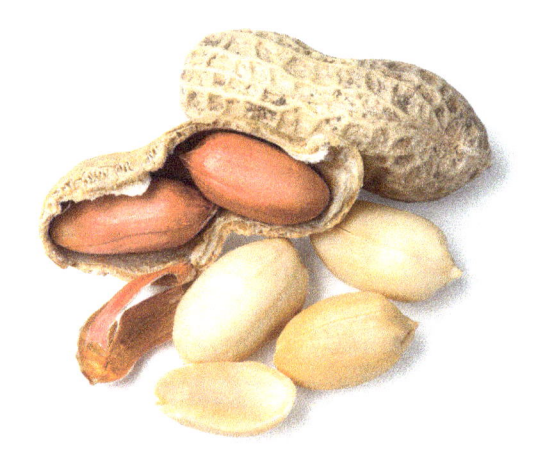

Modern Tradition

Good source of fiber, aids in digestion, and excellent source of biotin.

#25–POTATO

Ancient Wisdom: Inexpensive and well-balanced nutrient.

Flavor: Sweet
Temperature: Neutral, slightly cold
Function:
    Treats hepatitis, stomach ulcers, and tonsilitis
Organ System: SP, ST

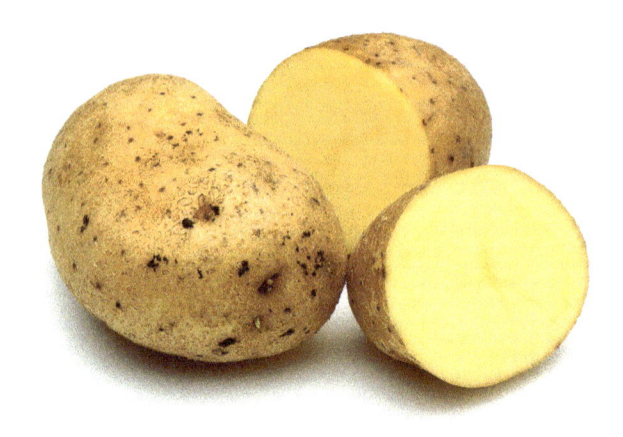

Modern Tradition

It has rich amino acid and enormous potassium. It is a good medicine for treating indigestion. It is more nutritious than rice or wheat. If you eat 250 grams a day, you would have enough vitamins to support you for a day and night. It is considered to be a perfect nutritious food in the eyes of nutritionists. Lowers cholesterol and improves heart health. Rich in vitamin C and fiber.

#26–RABBIT

Ancient Wisdom: The vegetarian meat.

Flavor: Sweet
Temperature: Cool
Function:
    Tonifies QI and yin

*100 grams of rabbit meat contains only 0.4 grams of fat, but 21.5 grams of protein. Only 1/7 of chicken meat, 1/25 of beef, and 1/50 of pork.

Organ System: LI, LV, SP, ST

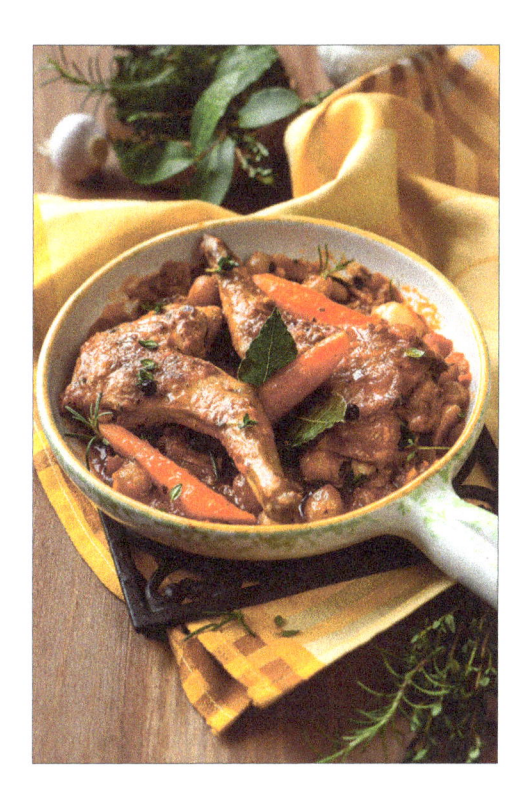

Modern Tradition

Excellent source of iron and contains vitamin G.

#27–RADISH
ANTI-CANCER FOOD

Ancient Wisdom: Also called "red turnips" due to the color and "pretty ginseng." Listed as "the vegetable of the nation" by the Dutch. The long life of the Japanese has everything to do with the consumption of this.

Flavor: Acrid, sweet
Temperature: Cool
Function:
- Brightens the eyes
- Clears heat
- Dissolves the stagnation of QI or food
- Good for people of all ages
- Improves immunity
- Transforms phlegm
- Treats bloating, cough, diabetes, migraines, and nosebleeds
- Can strengthen the spleen (per TCM)
- Tonifies deficiency

Organ System: LI, ST

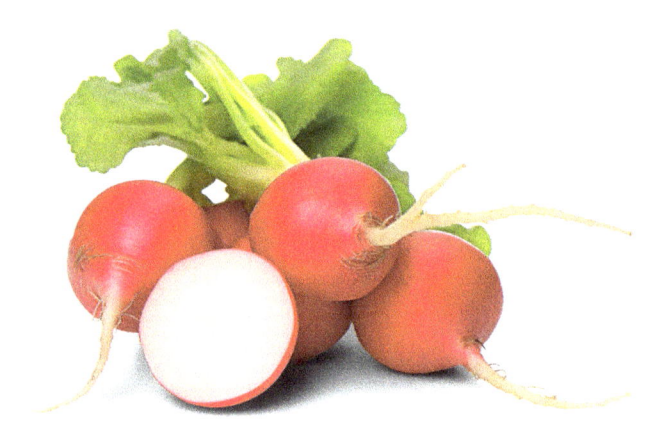

Modern Tradition

Contains vitamin C, potassium, can lower blood pressure, promote the generation of collagen, and prevents diabetes.

#28–RICE

Ancient Wisdom:

Flavor: Sweet
Temperature: Warm
Function:
    Stops diarrhea
    Treats spontaneous sweating
Organ System: SP, LU

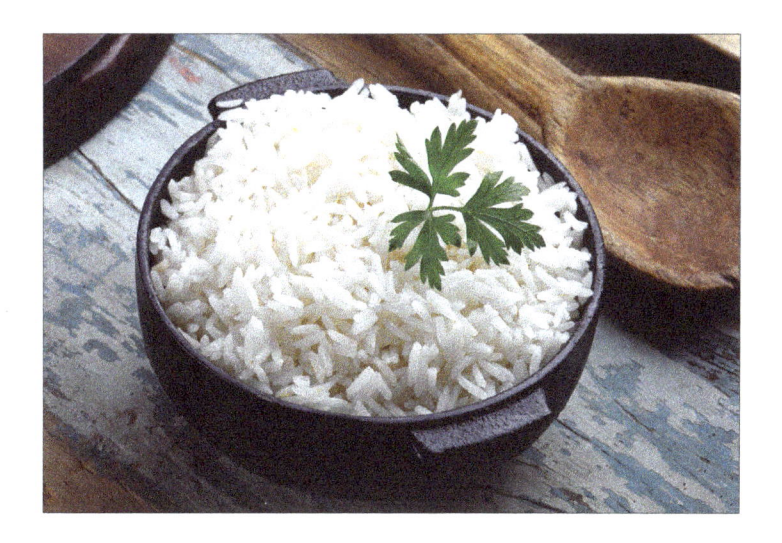

Modern Tradition

White rice restores glycogen levels post exercise.

#29–ROYAL JELLY
ANTI-CANCER FOOD

Ancient Wisdom: First choice for liver problems.

Flavor: Sweet
Temperature: Neutral
Function:
- Anti-cancer elements
- Builds the blood
- Helps with digestion
- Protects the liver
- Reduces fatigue
- Treats insomnia

*The queen bee can live for more than five years while ordinary working bees can live for only three months.

Organ System: LV, SP

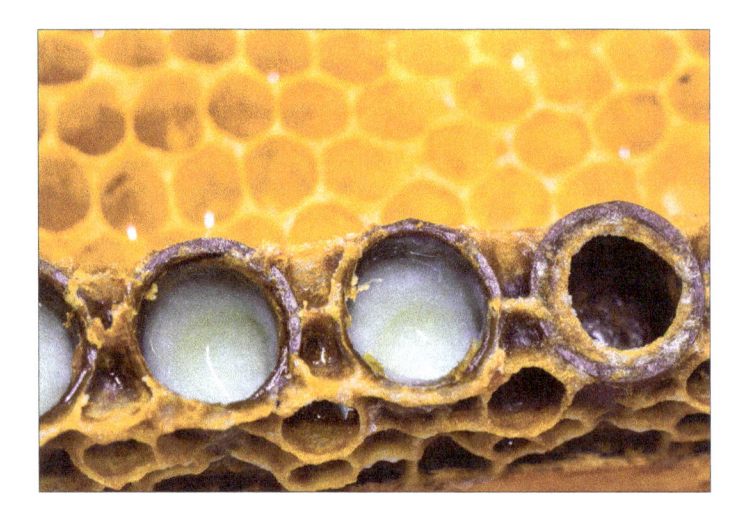

Modern Tradition

Treats neurodegenerative disorders, antibiotic, protective effects on reproductive health, enhances collagen, and eases premenstrual and post-menopausal symptoms.

#30–SESAME SEEDS

Ancient Wisdom: Eat 20 grams daily after breakfast.

Flavor: Sweet
Temperature: Neutral
Function:
    A traditional anti-anging nutrient
    Moistens the intestines
    Promotes lactation
    Returns hair to normal color
    Rich in vitamin
    Strengthens the spleen
    Tonifies the blood
    Treats constipation and paralysis in the legs
    Treats vertigo

*According to Stories of the Immortals, A Woman named Lu could still walk for 300 li daily as fast as a deer in her eighties. When asked for the secret, she said she had been eating sesame cakes all her life.

Organ System: KD, LI, LU, LV

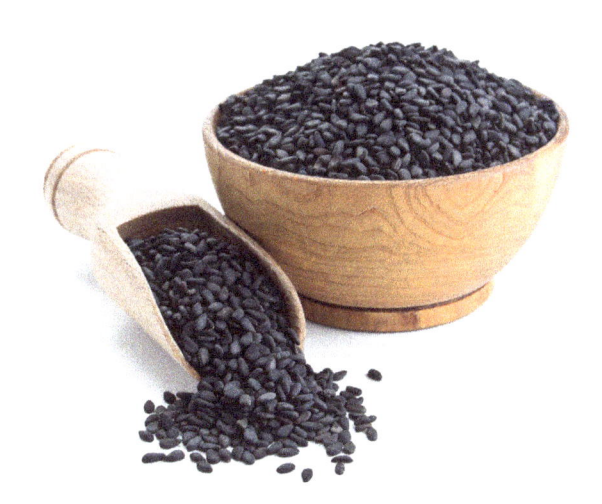

Modern Tradition

Lowers blood pressure and blood sugar. Promotes healthy thyroid function, brain health, and energy levels. Improves digestion. Prevents diabetes.

#31–SHAN ZHA / HAWTHORN
ANTI-CANCER FOOD

Ancient Wisdom:

Flavor: Sour, sweet
Temperature: Warm
Function:
  Acts as a diuretic
  Benefits digestion
  Expels blood stasis
  Detoxicates
  Dissolves phlegm
  Reduces body fat
  Reduces high blood pressure

Organ System: HT-LV-SP-ST

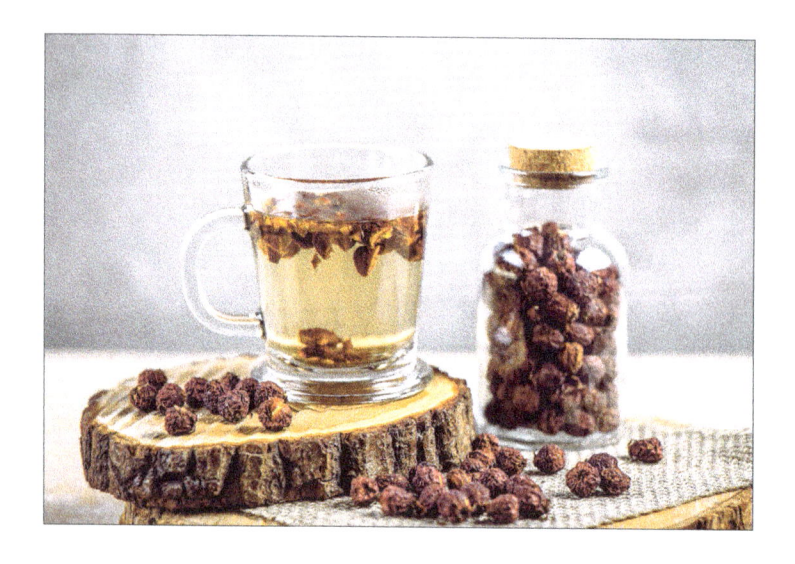

Modern Tradition

Hawthorn improves blood flow and dilates blood vessels, regulates blood pressure, lowers cholesterol, aids in digestion, and reduces anxiety. Anti-aging food and helps to prevent heart failure.

#32–SOYBEANS

Ancient Wisdom: Top of the list of all beans.

Flavor: Sweet
Temperature: Cool, neutral
Function:
    Eliminates constipation, diarrhea, and toxins
    Slows down bleeding form injury
    Tonifies the qi and blood
    Treats iron-based anemia
    Treats edema, leg ulcers, morning sickness, renal failure, and toxemia during pregnancy

*Every 100 grams of soy beans contains 36.3 grams of protein and 18.4 grams of fat. Top on the list of all beans.

Organ System: LI, SP, ST

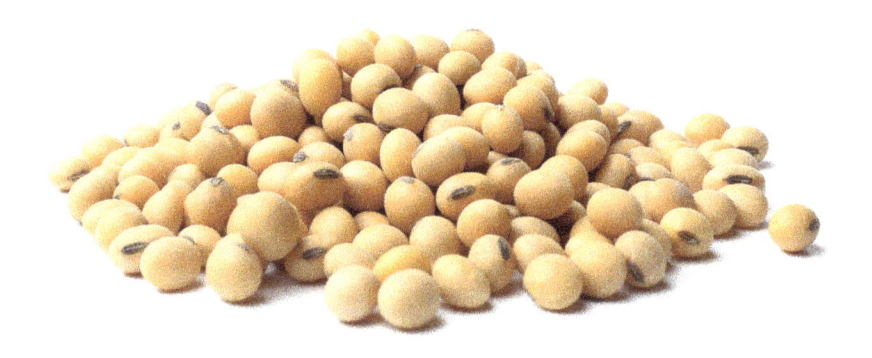

Modern Tradition

Reduces risk of stroke, cardiovascular disease, coronary heart disease, promotes heart health, and improves bone health.

#33–SPINACH

Ancient Wisdom: Good for people with hypertension and diabetes.

Flavor: Sweet
Temperature: Cool
Function:
> Helps to treat and prevent nosebleeds, constipation, and diabetes
> Rich in iron, protein, and vitamins
> Reduces gastric juice secretion and secretion of the pancreas
> Restores the malfunctioning of the stomach and reparatory system
> Tonifies blood and yin

Organ System: LI, LV, ST

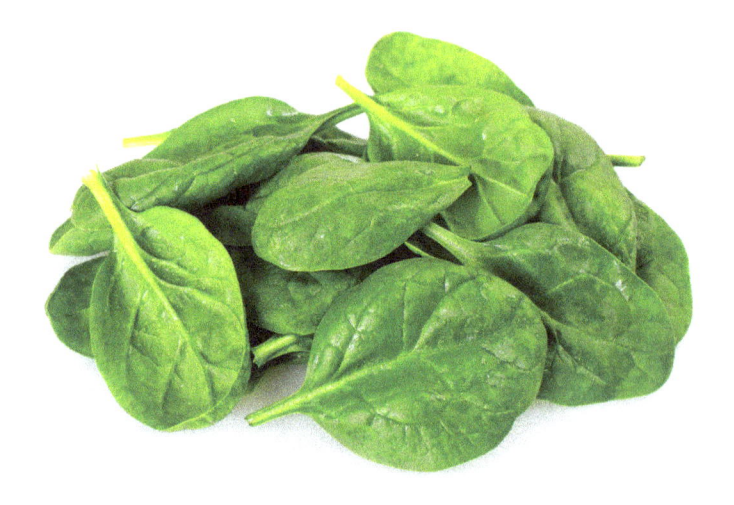

Modern Tradition

Supports brain health, helps maintain healthy blood pressure, and improves eye health.

#34–TOMATO
ANTI-CANCER FOOD

Ancient Wisdom: Lots of vitamins C, PP, and D.

Flavor: Sweet, sour
Temperature: Cold
Function:
- Clears heat
- Good for diabetes
- Eliminates toxins
- Helps dizziness
- Stops thirst
- Tonifies yin
- Treats mouth sores

Organ System: LV, ST

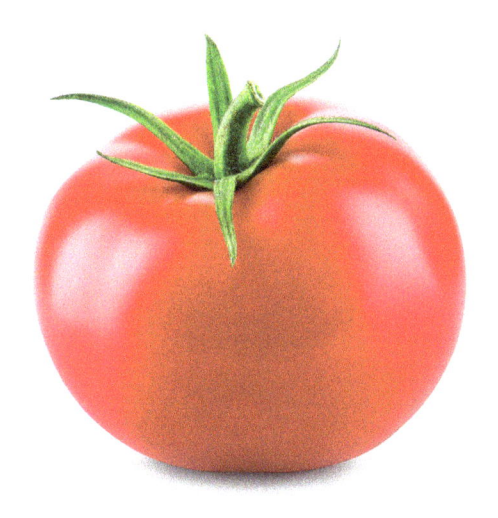

Modern Tradition

Contains lycopene, which has anti-cancer properties. Reduces insulin resistance and lowers risk of severe depression and cholesterol.

#35–WALNUTS

Ancient Wisdom:
Long life nut. In ancient Russia, it was called "food of the strong men."

Flavor: Sweet
Temperature: Warm
Function:
    Treats frequent urination
    Impotence
    Strengthens kidneys
    Tonifies the brain and liver
Organ System: KD, LI, LU

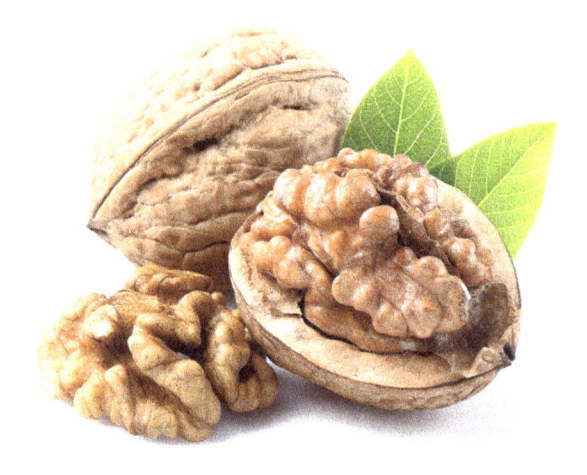

Modern Tradition

Rich in omega-3, anti-inflammatory, promotes gut health, promotes weight loss, and lowers blood pressure.

#36–WATERMELON

Ancient Wisdom:

Flavor: Sweet
Temperature: Cold
Function:
- Clears heat
- Disinhibits urination
- Good for mouth sores and sore throat
- Helps to prevent and treat stroke
- Prevents constipation
- Protects against cancer in the esophagus

Organ System: BL, HT, ST

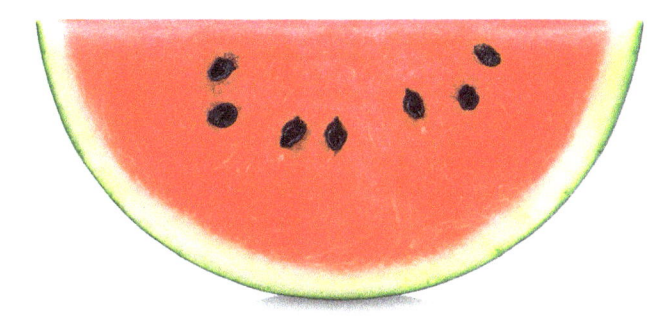

Modern Tradition

Contains lycopene, aids digestion, helps maintain hydration, promotes weight loss, improves heart health and treats UTI.

SECTION II

W.O.W. QUIZ

World of Wisdom

Identify how to strengthen your organ systems to optimize your health.

Instructions:

Answer "Yes" or "No" to each of the following questions below.
Don't worry about what the symptoms mean; just note whether or not you experience them.

Once you are finished, tally your score separately for each section. Note which section you have the most "Yes's" in. This is the organ system for you which is likely to be the most imbalanced. See the list of foods after the test support that organ system and put them on your grocery list to help improve your condition.

*Important Note: This is not a medical exam, nor is it considered to be a medical assessment. To be adequately and accurately assessed for you own personal, differential, and optimized food therapy prescription, you must see a highly trained acupuncturist or doctor of acupuncture and oriental medicine.

Kidney

1. Do you have soreness, weakness, or pain in lower back or knee?
2. Do you have buzzing in your ears or experience dizziness?
3. Is your hair prematurely gray, or do you have dark circles around or underneath your eyes?
4. Do you have night sweats or hot flashes?
5. Would you describe yourself as afraid a lot?
6. Does your tongue lack coating?
    *Note: Always evaluate before you brush your teeth or eat.
7. Does your mouth, throat, or eyes often feel dry?
8. Do you wake up during the night and have difficulty falling back to sleep?
9. Are your feet cold, especially at night, or are you typically colder than those around you?
10. Is your libido low?

Gallbladder

1. Do you have muscle and body pain?
2. Do you have difficulty making decisions?
3. Do you experience dizziness or vertigo?
4. Do you have trouble being assertive or following through with your plans?
5. Do you get migraines or headaches sometimes in the back of your head?
6. Do you have deafness, difficulty hearing, or tinnitus (a buzzing in your ears)?
7. Do you have a lack of confidence and/or feel timid or uninspired?
8. Do you struggle with digestive issues?
9. Do have or have had gallstones?
10. Do you sometimes have hypochondriac distention (a feeling of fullness under your ribs)?

Heart

1. Do you have difficulty falling asleep (insomnia)?
2. Do you feel anxious, depressed, and restless? Do you sometimes feel mental tiredness or are easily startled?
3. Do you have poor memory?
4. Do you experience palpitations?
5. Do you experience shortness of breath upon exertion?
6. Do you sweat easily/ more than others?
7. Do you often have vivid dreams?
8. Do you have tongue ulcers?
9. Are you prone to motion sickness?
10. Have you been diagnosed with schizophrenia or SLE?

Liver

1. Do you have eye problems?
2. Do your muscles cramp easily and get stiff?
3. Do you have tingling or numbness in your toes or fingers?
4. Do you get dizzy?
5. Do you tend to sigh often and/or have a bitter taste in your mouth?
6. Do you have a lump in your throat, but the doctors can't find anything?
7. Do you have clots in your menses or have breast distention?
8. Do you anger easily or experience moodiness?
9. Do you feel bloated after you eat?
10. Do you sigh frequently and feel irritable?

Spleen

1. Do you tire easily, or commonly catch colds or viruses?
2. Do you feel worried a lot and overthink?
3. Do you tend to have loose stools?
4. Do you have a sallow complexion?
5. Do you have a poor or reduced appetite?
6. Do you feel fullness in your abdomen?
7. Do you have or have you had prolapse (e.g., anus, protruding hemorrhoids, stomach, uterus, vagina)?
8. Do you experience frequent, urgent urination, and/or sometimes leak urine?
9. Do you have weakness in your limbs or feel a heaviness?
10. Do you have white vaginal discharge?

Stomach

1. Do you have GERD or acid reflux?
2. Do you burp often or regurgitate?
3. Do you have stomach pain in your abdomen?
4. Do you get hungry easily?
5. Do you have a strong appetite?
6. Do you have bleeding gums?
7. Do you get stomach pain that feels better after you vomit or have a bowel movement?
8. Do you feel nauseous often?
9. Does your tongue have a thick white or yellow coating?
10. Do you have foul breath?

Lung

1. Do you experience shortness of breath, which becomes worse upon exertion?
2. Do you sweat during the day for no apparent reason?
3. Do you have skin problems?
4. Do you feel sad more than anything else?
5. Do you have phlegm in your throat or feel like you always have to cough?
6. Do you tend to have a dry throat, hoarse voice, and/or dry skin?
7. Do you lack the desire to talk?
8. Do you have a pale white complexion?
9. Do people say you look like you are cold?
10. Do you have a taste of metal in your mouth?

Instructions: Tally your score separately for each section. Note which section you have the most 'Yes'. This is the Organ system for you which is the likely to be the most imbalanced. See below which foods support that organ system and put them on your grocery list to help improve your condition.

FOODS THAT BENEFIT YOUR ORGANS

GALLBLADDER:
Barley
Corn

HEART:
Adzuki Beans
Alcohol
Bamboo Shoots
Beet
Bitter Melon
Cantaloupe
Chestnut
Coffee
Eggplant
Ginger
Green Tea
Green Pepper
Hawthorn Fruit
Hearts
Honeydew Melon
Lotus Seeds
Mushrooms
Noodles
Nuts
Persimmons
Red Pepper
Soy Beans
Watermelon
Wheat

KIDNEY:
Abalone
Asparagus
Bamboo Shoots
Beef
Black Sesame Seeds
Black Beans
Black Soy Beans

Bone Broth
Carp Fish
Chestnut
Chinese Yam
Chive
Clams
Coffee
Cuddle Fish
Duck
Goji Berries
Grapes
Kelp
Kidney Beans
Lamb
Lotus Seeds
Miso
Oyster
Plum
Pork
Seaweed
String Beans
Sweet Potato
Tangerine
Walnut
Warm Water
Wheat
Wild Rice (in-moderation)

LARGE INTESTINE:
Agar
Alfalfa Sprouts
Almond,
Apple
Apricot
Bamboo Shoots
Banana
Beef
Black Fungus

Black Pepper
Broccoli
Cantaloupe
Carp Fish
Cauliflower
Chinese Cabbage
Cabbage
Cornbread
Cucumber
Eggplant
Green Tea
Honey
Honeydew Melon
Lettuce
Persimmons
Spinach
Tofu
Watermelon "Dong Gua"
White Pepper
Yellow Soy Bean

LIVER
Abalone
Alcohol
Beef
Beet
Black Sesame Seeds
Brown Sugar
Carrots
Celery
Chicken
Chives
Clams
Coffee
Crab Meat
Cuddle Fish
Eel
Hawthorne Fruit

Green Tea
Leek
Liver
Lychee
Red Wine
Royal Jelly
Sour Plum
Vinegar

LUNG:
Agar
Alcohol
Almond
Apple
Apricot
Asparagus
Bamboo Shoots
Banana
Bok Choy
Cantaloupe
Carrots
Cinnamon Twig
Coffee
Duck Meat
Garlic
Ginger
Grapes
Green Tea
Honey
Honeydew Melon
Leek
Milk
Peanuts
Pears
Peppermint
Radish
Sugarcane
Tangerine
Walnuts

SMALL INSTESTINE:
Adzuki Beans
Cantaloupe
Honeydew Melon

SPLEEN:
Alfalfa Sprouts
Almonds
Apples
Apricot
Asparagus
Avocado
Barley
Beef
Berries
Bone Broth
Broccoli
Cabbage
Carrot
Chicken
Cinnamon
Clams
Coconut Oil
Congee
Ginger
Goji Berries
Lamb
Lentils
Millet
Miso Soup
Nutmeg
Oats
Olive Oil
Orange Peels
Plum
Poultry
Pumpkin
Quinoa
Root Vegetables
Salmon
Squash
Sunflower Seeds

Sweet Potato
Taro
Warm Water
Watermelon

STOMACH:
Alcohol
Alfalfa Sprouts
Apple
Apricot
Bamboo Shoots
Barley
Beef
Bean Curd
Beef
Bitter Melon
Black Fungus
Black Soy Beans
Bok Choy
Broccoli
Cabbage
Carp Fish
Carrots
Celery
Chicken
Clams
Coffee
Crab
Cucumber
Eggplant
Garlic
Ginger
Grapes
Green Tea
Hawthorn Fruit
Lettuce
Peanuts
Plum
Pork
Rice
Salt
Squash

Vinegar Wine
Watermelon
Wheat
White Sugar
Yellow Soy Beans
Yi Yi Ren

URINARY BLADDER:
Bok Choy
Broccoli
Cantaloupe
Chinese Dong Gua
Cinnamon Bark
Cinnamon Twig
Fish (Wild)
Grapes
Green Tea
Honeydew Melon
Plum
Watermelon

FOODS THAT BENEFIT VARIOUS MEDICAL CONDITIONS

ADHD:
Bamboo Shoots
Exercise
Fresh Fruits
Fresh Vegetables
Vitamin B Complex

ADRENALS:
Bamboo Shoots

ALZHEIMERS / COGNITIVE DECLINE / DEMENTIA:
Apple
Berries
Black Beans
Celery
Chaga Mushroom
Chickpeas
Coconut Oil
Cordyceps
Fiber
Flavonoids
Fresh Fruit
Fresh Vegetables
Garlic
Kidney Beans
Leafy Greens
Legumes
Lemon
Lime
Lion's Mane
Mushrooms
Onions
Oyster Mushrooms
Radish
Reishi
Saffron
Shitake
Soybeans
Vitamin B1
Walnuts

*__Note:__ Eat plenty of organic fresh fruits, fresh vegetables, and fiber. Alleviate AGEs, dairy, endotoxins, gluten, glycol-toxins, meat, saturated fat, sugar. Avoid aluminum, copper, fluoride, heavy metals, iron, and pesticides. Avoid a high cholesterol diet. Use lemon balm for aromatherapy.

ANEMIA:
Asparagus
Barley
Beef
Beets
Black Sesame Seed
Egg
Liver
Pork
Rabbit
Squid

ANTI-CANCER FOODS:

Asparagus	Ginger	Radish
Bamboo Shoots	Green Tea	Shitake
Black Fungus	Hawthorn Fruit	Spinach
Burdock Root	Honey	Tomato
Corn	Kelp	Watermelon
Cucumber	Lotus Seeds	
Garlic	Onion	

ANXIETY:

Asparagus	Celery	Chia Seeds
Black Sesame Seeds	Chamomile	Chinese Dates
Goat Milk	Lemon	Orange
Goji Berries	Lime	
Leafy Green	Lotus Seeds	

APPETITE (IMPROVES):

Bamboo Shoots	Fava Bean	Shitake
Chicken	Lotus Seeds	
Chives	Red Date	

ARTERIOSCLEROSIS:

Avocado	Chestnuts	Green Tea
Beets	Citrus	Lemon
Berries	Cranberries	Spinach
Blueberries	Flaxseeds	Tomato
Cabbage	Garlic	Walnuts
Celery	Grapefruit	

ARTHRITIS:

Chestnuts

ASTHMA:

Apple	Ginkgo Seeds	Radish
Apricot Seeds	Leek	Spinach
Banana	Mango	Sunflower Seeds
Buckwheat	Mushroom	Turmeric
Fennel	Mustard Green	White Turnip
Garlic	Onions	
Ginger	Pumpkin	

BACK PAIN (LOW):

Beef	Chestnuts
Black Beans	Cinnamon

BLOATING:

Chives	Molasses	Pineapple

BLOOD PRESSURE:

Asparagus	Chestnut	Oats
Banana	Corn	Onions
Beets	Flaxseed	Pineapple
Black Beans	Garlic	Quinoa
Black Sesame Seeds	Goji Berry	b
Blueberries	Hawthorn Fruit	Spinach
Celery	Legumes	

BLOOD SUGAR (STABILIZES):
Asparagus

BLURRED VISION:

Black Sesame Seeds	Goji Berry
Eggs	Longan

BREAST ABSCESSES:
Eggplant

BRAIN HEALTH:

Black Sesame Seeds	Grapes	Walnuts
Celery	Mushrooms	
Ginger	Protein	

BRUISES:
Chestnuts

CATARACTS:

Abalone	Fresh Vegetables	Sweet Potato
Chrysanthemum Tea	Goji Berries	

CHOLESTEROL:

Artichoke	Bergamot	Celery
Bamboo Shoots	Black Beans	
Banana	Brazil Nuts	

RASBERRIES
Red Yeast Rice

CHEST PAIN:

Cabbage	Mustard Greens	Saffron

COLON HEALTH:
Black Beans

CONSTIPATION:

Asparagus	Cabbage	Pear
Bamboo Shoots	Cantaloupe	Pine Nut
Banana	Honeydew Melon	Pumpkin Seeds
Beets	Muskmelon	Spinach
Black Beans	Peas	Sweet Potato

CORONARY DISEASE:
Chestnuts

COUGH:
Abalone	Asparagus	Carrot

WHOOPING:
Garlic	Goji Berry	Mango

DRY COUGH:
Abalone	Honeydew Melon	Muskmelon
Cantaloupe	Lemon	Pine Nut
Eggs	Molasses	

DEPRESSION:
Banana	Legumes	Walnuts
Berries	Salmon	
Broccoli	Turmeric	

DETOXIFY:
Bamboo	Cauliflower	Fennel
Black Beans	Collard Greens	Kale
Broccoli	Cruciferous Vegetables	Radish
Brussel Sprouts	Dandelion	Scallion
Cabbage	Eggplant	

DIABETES:
Almond	Beef	Green Beans
Asparagus	Celery	Sweet Potato
Avocado	Garlic	
Barley	Goji Berry	

DIARRHEA:

Barley	Green Beans	Olives
Carrot	Green Tea	Onions
Chicken	Hazelnut	Rice
Cinnamon	Litchi	Sweet Potato
Coconut	Millet	Red Dates
Fava Beans	Mung Bean	
Garlic	Nutmeg	

DIGESTION:

Banana	Cauliflower	Peas
Barley	Chives	Pineapple
Black Beans	Lemon	Plum
Carrot	Mango	

DIZZINESS:

Goji Berry	Pine Nut	Strawberries
Green Tea	Saffron	
Longan	Sesame Seeds	

DOWNS SYNDROME:

Chinese Yam	Cinnamon

ECZEMA:
INGEST:

Berries	Green Tea	Radish
Broccoli	Herring	Salmon
Celery	Kale	Sardines
Citrus	Kimchi	Turmeric
Coconut Oil	Kombucha	Vitamin B Complex
Fresh Fruits	Leafy Greens	Zinc
Fresh Vegetables	Miso	
	Oolong Tea	

TOPICAL:

Coconut Oil	Primrose Oil	Hemp Seed Oil

AVOID:

Chicken	Eggs	Milk

EDEMA:

Barley	Fava Beans	Kidney Beans
Chicken	Ginger	Peas
Coconut	Hawthorn Fruit	

EYE HEALTH:

Abalone	Carrot	Hazelnut
Black Beans	Eggs	
Broccoli	Goji Berry	

FATIGUE:

Almonds	Cinnamon	Quinoa
Banana	Flaxseeds	Red Date
Barley	Green Tea	Royal Jelly
Black Beans	Hazelnut	Shitake
Black Sesame Seeds	Litchi	Strawberry
Cherries	Molasses	Sweet Potato
Chia Seeds	Oatmeal	
Chicken	Pumpkin	

FOOT WEAKNESS:

Kelp	Pineapple

FREQUENT URINATION:

Chicken	Raspberry

GALLSTONES:

Corn

GINGIVITIS/ BLEEDING GUMS:
Plum

HAIR LOSS (ALOPECIA):
Adzuki Beans	Grapes	Potato
Asparagus	Kelp	Raisins
Black Beans	Kidney Beans	Rice
Black Sesame Seeds	Lemon	String Beans
Chinese Yam	Lime	Sweet Potato
Goji Berries	Mulberries	

HAND WEAKNESS:
Pineapple

HANGOVER:
Olive   Strawberry

HEADACHE:
Basil   Green Tea

HEART HEALTH:
Bamboo Shoots	Celery	Longan
Banana	Chestnut	Lotus Seed

HEMORRHOIDS:
Chestnut	Onion	Spinach
Eggplant	Pumpkin Seeds	Turtle
Lotus Seeds	Radish	Water
Milk	Seaweed	
Mushrooms	Sesame Seeds	

HEMOPTYSIS:
Asparagus

HEMORRHOIDS:
Adzuki Beans

HEPATITIS:
Corn

HOARSE VOICE:
Chicken

HORMONES–REGULATES:
Bamboo Shoots

INFERTILITY:
Black Beans

IMMUNITY:
Asparagus   Bamboo Shoots

IMPOTENCE:
Goji Berry   Shrimp

INSOMNIA:
Chamomile Tea   Longan

JAUNDICE:
Adzuki Beans   Barley   Corn

KIDNEY FAILURE:
Bamboo Shoots

KNEE PAIN:
Beef   Cinnamon
Black Beans   Goji Berry

LACTATION:

Chicken	Peanuts	Shrimp
Lettuce	Pumpkin Seeds	

MEDICINE TOXICITY:
Mung Bean

MEMORY:

Celery	Longan

MENSTRUAL IRREGULARITIES:
Beets

MOUTH SORES:

Goat Milk	Plum

NAUSEA:

Green Bean	Mango

NEUROLOGICAL DISORDERS:
Celery

NOSE BLEEDS:

Chestnut	Lotus Root	Spinach

PAIN (REDUCE) (RICH IN GLUTATHION)

Asparagus	Cottage Cheese	Wild Caught Fish (Cod, Tuna, Salmon)
Bone Broth	Grass-Fed Beef	Turkey
Broccoli Rabe	Spirulina/ KOMBU	Venison
Chinese Cabbage		

PAIN:
Pumpkin

PALPITATIONS:
Longan					Lotus Seeds

PARALYSIS:
Cherry

PREGNANCY HEALTH:
Asparagus

PREMATURE EJACULATION:
Sweet Potato				Lotus Seeds

RED EYES:
Tomato

RENAL REPERFUSION:
Bamboo Shoots

RESTLESSNESS:
Lotus Seed				Red Date

SEMINAL EMISSIONS:
Black Beans				Lotus Seeds
Green Beans				Raspberry

SHORTNESS OF BREATH:
Red Date				Shitake

SPERMATORRHEA:
Goji Berry

SPONTANEOUS SWEATS:
Oats

STOMACH ACHE:
Litchi

STOMACH ULCER:
Banana

TAPEWORM:
Coconut

TESTOSTERONE:

Almonds	Coffee	Macadamia Nut
Asparagus	Dairy Products	Milk
Avocado	Eggs	Olive Oil (Extra Virgin)
Banana	Fatty Fish	*Onion
Brazil Nuts	Fatty Oil	Oysters
Beans	*Flavonoids	Parsley
Black Beans	Garlic	Pomegranate
Blue Cheese	Honey	Pumpkin Seeds
*Broccoli	*Hot Peppers	Raisins
Cabbage	*Kale	*Rutabaga
Cacao (Raw)	Kidney Beans	*Spinach
Cauliflower	Leafy Greens	Sweet Potato
Cereals (Fortified)	Lemon	Tuna
Chia Seeds	Legumes	Walnuts
Coconut	Maca Root	Yogurt

THYROID:
Bamboo Shoots

URINARY PROBLEMS:

Abalone	Corn	Peas
Adzuki Beans	Fava Beans	Pineapple
Barley	Green Bean	Plum
Broccoli	Green Tea	Raspberries

Cantaloupe	Honeydew Melon	Watermelon
Celery	Lettuce	
Coconut	Muskmelon	

UTI:
Abalone	Adzuki Beans	Watermelon

VAGINAL BLEEDING:
Abalone	Chicken

VAGINAL DISCHARGE:
Abalone	Chicken	Green Bean

VERTIGO:
Celery	Sesame Seeds

WEIGHT LOSS:
Apple	Cucumber	Oats
Asparagus	Eggs	Onions
Avocado	Flax Seeds	Oolong Tea
Banana	Garlic	Radish
Blueberries	Ginger Root	Salmon
Broccoli	Green Tea	Shitake
Carrots	Liver	Sweet Potato
Celery	Lotus Seed	Walnuts
Chestnuts	Millet	Water
Chicken	Mung Beans	Watermelon
Cinnamon	Mulberry Fruit	

WORMS:
Onions	Pumpkin Seed

SECTION III

ASK DR. LIZ

ASK DR. LIZ #1

ACUPUNCTURE

Q: What is acupuncture?
A: Acupuncture is a part of oriental medicine known as Traditional Chinese Medicine (TCM). It is one of the oldest and most effective medical systems in the world when it comes to both preventing and treating chronic disease. Both TCM and ayurvedic medicine stem from pre-Qin Taoist thought. Acupuncture uses very thin needles that are strategically placed and scientifically based to balance the body into health.

Q: How can acupuncture help me?
A: Acupuncture can help prevent and treat many diseases, both chronic and acute, and can even help in trauma-based medical situations.

Q: Does the National Institute of Health (NIH) or the World Health Organization (WHO) support acupuncture and oriental medicine?
A: Yes. Both strongly support the use of acupuncture and oriental medicine for many diseases. In order to achieve best health results, it is often best to use both Western medicine alongside of TCM.

Q: What if I'm afraid of needles? Does it hurt to get acupuncture?
A: In many cases, you cannot even feel the needle! It is such an amazing medicine that you feel so good after a treatment, the small amount of occasional discomfort it may possibly create is minimal in terms of its many benefits. Many acupuncturists are trained to safely and effectively prescribe you with herbal decoctions, as well, and not use needles.

Q: Are acupuncturists doctors?
A: Acupuncturists go through extensive medical training. They study internal medicine extensively. Acupuncture physicians are trained in anatomy and physiology, biochemistry, pathophysiology, and boarded in acupuncture, biomedicine, herbology, and traditional medicine. Many are certified with NCCAOM. Further, they are trained in organ system meridian pathways which is how and why an acupuncturist can effectively help treat numerous diseases so effectively.[1]

Q: Who should go for acupuncture?
A: Everyone should! It's super healthy and excellent for prevention as well as treatment. It is best to go to a NCCAOM certified and licensed acupuncture physician (AP) or diplomate of oriental

medicine (DOM) to receive acupuncture. Acupuncture physicians (AP) are far more educated in treating you using acupuncture than a chiropractor, medical doctor (MD) or physical therapist (PT).

Q: What do you go to acupuncture for?
A: Acupuncture helps improve so many medical conditions from anemia, fertility, headaches, menopause, pain, and much more. I had post-concussive syndrome and experienced anxiety, balance issues, dizziness, fatigue, and intermittent brain bleeds. This went on for months and it was debilitating.

Q: How many acupuncture treatments did you receive?
A: Fourteen. Natural herbs and acupuncture were both prescribed by my TCM doctor. After the first treatment, I felt measurably better! Within a month's period, my problem was fully resolved. I became a believer in acupuncture and custom herbal therapeutics ever since.

Q: My mother has Parkinson's disease and my aunt has colitis and cancer. Can acupuncture and oriental medicine help with that?[2]
A: Indeed, it can, and very effectively.

ASK DR. LIZ #2

ALCOHOL

Q: Should we consume alcohol?
A: Everyone agrees that heavy alcohol consumption, binge drinking, and any alcohol during pregnancy is bad. However, studies do show that consuming one to two drinks a day can be helpful for the average American. Moderate consumption of alcohol can reduce the risk of a heart attack and is shown to decrease our risk of the "clotting" type of stroke, but it does increase our risk of cancer and a "bleeding" kind of stroke.

Q: Who benefits most from "moderate" alcohol intake?
A: The answer is the "average" American. For the "healthy" person, this means anyone who exercises thirty minutes or more per day, doesn't smoke, and eats at least one serving of fruits or vegetables per day. In this study, this is what is defined as a "healthy" person or a "health freak" in America. According to this study, one to two drinks per day provided no benefit to the "healthy" American.

Q: What about alcohol and breast cancer?
A: There is convincing evidence that moderate alcohol intake does increase the chances of having breast cancer.

Q: What about heavy consumption of alcohol and breast cancer?
A: Even consumption of less than a single alcoholic beverage per day results in carcinogenic concentrations of acetaldehyde produced from the alcohol in the oral cavity. Even mouthwash that contains alcohol can give you a carcinogenic spike. So, surely prudent public health policy pertaining to breast cancer would recommend to avoid alcohol consumption at all, let alone heavy alcohol consumption.

Q: What is the number one killer for women in the United States? Is it breast cancer?
A: The number one killer in the U.S. for women is heart disease, not breast cancer. Studies do show that one to two drinks per day do promote health in general for the "average" American, even though alcohol is shown to increase the risk of breast cancer in women in any amount.

Q: What is the risk for women who have already been diagnosed with breast cancer?
A: Women can cut their risk in half of dying just by consuming five or more servings of fruits and vegetables daily and walking thirty minutes per day, six days per week, and not drinking any alcohol.

Q: What is the number one thing anyone can do to prevent cancer of any kind?
A: Eat more daily servings of both fruits and vegetables.

Q: What about grapes in the wine that we drink? Are they good for us?
A: Interestingly, red grapes, specifically the ones with seeds that are used to make red wine, do have health benefits and are shown to better protect the body and prevent cancer. The white grapes just don't do it.[3]

ASK DR. LIZ #3

LET'S PREVENT ALZHEIMER'S

Q: Tell me about Alzheimer's disease and how to prevent it?
A: Alzheimer's is the fastest growing disease in America, and you are wise to inquire about prevention.

Q: I'm over sixty years old. Is it still effective to practice some of these protocols?
A: Yes. It's never too late to make smart lifestyle changes!

Q: What are some scientifically proven ways I can help improve brain function and prevent Alzheimer's disease?
A: I will share with you eight different ways you can start to prevent this disease:

1. Fruits and vegetables
2. Omega-3 fatty acids (DHA)
3. Prevent plaque on teeth
4. Avoid fluoride
5. Avoid aluminum
6. Avoid alcohol
7. Walk backwards for ten minutes/day
8. Take turmeric

Q: Should I eat salmon?
A: Yes! It is wise to increase your omega-3 fatty acids, which contain DHA. This is generally good food for the brain and its function. You can also enjoy tuna, sardines, and mackerel if you choose.

Q: What about the plaque on my teeth?
A: It is very important to keep your teeth and gums clean, plaque free, and healthy! If your body is prone to creating excess plaque, get your teeth cleaned more often. Perhaps a cleaning every three months is appropriate. Studies do show the relationship between plaque in the mouth and plaque in the brain is found to relate to Alzheimer's disease. So, if you keep plaque out of your mouth, you are more likely to keep the same plaque out of your brain![4]

Q: What about fluoride?
A: Fluoride is strongly suspected to be toxic to brain health. Numerous studies show that extremely high levels of fluoride are known to cause neurotoxicity in adults. Harvard School of Public Health found strong indications that fluoride may adversely affect cognitive development in children. This

was based on meta-analysis of twenty-seven studies. Although more research is warranted, you may consider staying away from fluoride in your toothpaste, mouthwash, and fluoride in your water.[5]

Q: What about aluminum?
A: It may be wise to avoid aluminum, as well. This includes touching foil or allowing foil products to touch your food. Small particles from the foil itself can attach themselves to your food and get into your bloodstream through digestion and potentially cause disease, possibly dementia or Alzheimer's disease. If you are freezing food and it is first wrapped in an inner layer of safe product, it is then okay to put foil around the preliminary layer, so long as it is not making any direct contact with your food.[6]

Q: What about the aluminum that can be found in deodorant?
A: Change to a deodorant that does not contain aluminum. You can search online or go to a health food store to find natural deodorants. Some work better than others in terms of their actual function. I personally recommend Alvera's all-natural roll-on deodorant, aloe and almonds.

Q: How about exercise?
A: Exercise is very important for overall good health! It is also key in preventing Alzheimer's. There are studies that show that walking backwards for ten minutes a day can help prevent and even reverse Alzheimer's disease! Please do this in a safe environment if you choose to try it.[7]

ASK DR. LIZ #4

AN APPLE A DAY

Q: Is it true an apple a day keeps the doctor away?
A: While it is still important to get regular checkups with your doctor, apples are loaded with antioxidants and very good for you!

Q: Is it important to eat the skin of the apple to receive these benefits?
A: Yes. There was a study done, evaluating the difference between peeled and unpeeled apples and the effect on suppressing cancer cells. The study showed that eating a standard red-skinned apple cut cancer cell rates over 50 percent![8]

Q: Which fruits fight cancer better?
A: In the study, liver cancer patients were utilized. Apples were found to drop cancer rates, cutting the cancer cell growth in half.

Q: Were any other fruits tested and shown to be stronger?
A: Yes, lemons and cranberries are the winners in terms of cutting cancer cell growth.[9]

Q: What other health benefits are derived from apples?
A: Apples are rich in antioxidants, flavonoids, and fiber. The phytonutrients and antioxidants found in apples may not only help reduce the risk of cancer, but also reduce the risk of developing high blood pressure, diabetes, and heart disease – America's number one killer! Apples help repair cell damage caused from oxidative stress that occurs in our DNA during normal cell activity.

Q: What are some of the other benefits "an apple a day" provides?
A: An apple won't entirely replace your toothbrush, but chewing an apple will promote whiter, healthier teeth while lowering levels of bacteria in the mouth and throughout the body. Apples are also shown to protect the brain, lowering rates of Alzheimer's disease and further protecting the brain against Parkinson's disease.

Q: What about gallbladder disease?
A: Interestingly, gallstones form when there is too much cholesterol in your bile to maintain a liquidity. So, yes, an apple a day will also help to prevent gallbladder disease and gallbladder stones.

Q: Anything else?
A: An apple a day can help to balance bowel activity including both diarrhea and constipation. The fiber in an apple can either help pull water out of your colon to manage loose stool or add water to the colon to effectively manage constipation or dry stools. An apple a day will generally help neutralize irritable bowel syndrome as well as avert hemorrhoids.

Q: What about eye diseases in the elderly?
A: Eating an apple a day is shown to lower the likelihood of cataracts by 10 to 15 percent!

ASK DR. LIZ #5

AVOCADO

Can Avocado Improve Cholesterol or Not?

Q: Are avocados healthy for me?
A: Yes, avocados are delicious, and offer some very definite health benefits. Avocados lower cholesterol, stabilize blood sugar, and are rich in potassium. They also lower small dense LDL cholesterol in our blood, which is the most dangerous type of cholesterol.

Q: What is it about avocadoes that makes them so unique?
A: Avocadoes are a type of a fruit. Adding them to a diet helps to lower small dense LDL cholesterol. The size distribution of the cholesterol becomes more benign, as well.[10]

Q: Do other foods help lower LDL cholesterol?
A: Yes, nuts and seeds are found to be beneficial, as well. Walnuts are excellent to help lower LDL cholesterol, too. Walnuts help keep your blood vessels healthy. Most nuts are healthy for your heart in general including hazelnuts, peanuts, almonds, and pistachios.

Q: Is all LDL cholesterol bad?
A: Yes. All LDL cholesterol is bad. Small dense LDL cholesterol is the worst!

Q: How do we prevent blood sugar and triglyceride spikes after meals?
A: Standard American meals lead to exaggerated spikes of sugar and fat in the blood, which generates oxidative stress inducing inflammation, and thickening of our blood. One bad meal can double your C-reactive protein (CRP)

Q: What is the best thing to do to avoid this?
A: A diet high in fiber, rich in fruits, vegetables, beans, sprouts, and avocadoes is the answer.

Q: Can nuts lessen insulin spikes?
A: Yes. Nuts can lessen sugar and insulin spikes. Almond butter after a bad meal or a handful of nuts can help lessen these spikes.

Q: What about the Avocado?
A: A half of an avocado can help stabilize blood sugar, too!

ASK DR. LIZ #6

GOING BANANAS?

Q: Is it true that 98 percent of American diets are potassium deficient?
A: Yes. Less than 2 percent of Americans achieve even the recommended minimum adequate intake of potassium due primarily to inadequate plant food intake.

Q: Does every cell in our body require potassium to function?
A: Yes, that is correct.

Q: How do we get more potassium in our diets?
A: It is best to eat more of a plant-based diet. Potassium is a mineral found in vegetables such as lima beans, Swiss chard, beet greens, sweet potatoes, soy beans, spinach, raisins, pinto beans, lentils, avocados, and, of course, bananas.

Q: Can I just take a potassium supplement?
A: It is best to eat fruits, vegetables, and nuts. Potassium supplements may cause diarrhea, irregular heartbeat, or mental confusion. Avoid taking potassium supplements if you have any form of kidney disease.

Q: What are the symptoms of low potassium?
A: A lower-than-normal amount of potassium in the blood is known as hypokalemia. Symptoms include problems with the GI tract, kidneys, muscles, heart, and nerves. A person may feel weakness, tiredness, or cramping in arm or leg muscles, tingling, muscle aches, or heart palpitations.

Q: Why don't we hear much about potassium from our doctors?
A: You don't hear much about potassium, but you should. It's important for muscle strength, nerve functioning, and a healthy cardiovascular system.

ASK DR. LIZ #7

ALZHEIMER'S AND CANDIDA

Q: Is there any relationship between Alzheimer's disease and Candida?
A: Yes. Recent findings show that the same plaque found in the brain of Alzheimer's disease patients is identical to the plaque *(amyloid beta)* found in Candida.

Q: How can I tell if I have Candida?
A: It's easy. First thing in the morning, spit into a glass of room temperature water. You must do this before you drink anything and before you brush your teeth. If the spit grows legs or sinks, you have Candida. If it floats on top, you likely don't. Give it about fifteen minutes total.

Q: What if I have Candida?
A: Most people in the United States do. The best way to eliminate Candida is to eat fresh fish, organic meat, plenty of organic fresh vegetables, alleviate gluten, sugar, dairy, and alcohol for at least six months. Then test again.

Q: If I do have Candida does that mean I am prone to Alzheimer's disease?
A: The dominant theory among researchers is that the plaque is the fundamental cause of Alzheimer's disease.

Q: What else can I do to find out if I am prone to Alzheimer's disease?
A: You can order a DNA test by going to 23andme.com. They will send you a packet in the mail. You must sign up for the health information.

Q: What must I do once I receive this kit?
A: You must spit into the capsule and mail it back to the self-addressed location. Within thirty days, they email you your personalized DNA strand, along with all kinds of information about your heritage, lineage, and global family members, which is fascinating.

Q: What do I do once I have this data?
A: You will find out your disease vulnerabilities. Some people are predisposed to AD and others are not. Your first goal should be to get rid of Candida.

ASK DR. LIZ #8

CELERY

Celery is the number one food for high blood pressure or hypertension. It is excellent for treating vertigo, Meniere's disease, headaches, dysentery, diarrhea with bloody stools, and chills and sweats. Celery strengthens the stomach and helps with urination. It tranquilizes the mind and is found to be good for people with poor nerves and arteriosclerosis. Celery calms down the liver, expels wind, and removes dampness.

Q: What vitamins and minerals does celery have in it?
A: Celery is an excellent vegetable that s healthy for the body for so many reasons. Celery is a source of vitamin K, potassium, dietary fiber, and manganese. It also is a very good source of vitamins B2, B6, and C, calcium, copper, phosphorous, and magnesium.

Q: Is it safe to eat the leaves of the celery stalk?
A: Yes. The leaves of the celery stalk contain a high content of vitamin A in the form of carotenoids.

Q: What are some of the other health benefits of celery?
A: Celery is the number one food for high blood pressure!

Q: What else does celery do for our health?
A: Celery helps rid constipation by promoting a smooth flow of bowel movement. It can treat dysentery with bloody stools and relieve chills and sweats. Consuming celery in your daily diet can also help relieve urinary problems. Celery can help you to relax, it's good for the liver, can help prevent and/or treat arteriosclerosis, and it's good for the nerves.

Q: What if you have stomach problems? Can you eat celery?
A: Yes. Celery strengthens the stomach.

Q: Can eating celery help with headaches?
A: Yes. Consuming celery can help with vertigo and headaches, too!

Q: What is the history of celery?
A: Celery was mentioned in Homer's *Odyssey* in and around 850 B.C. It was also recorded that celery leaves were found in the tomb of Pharaoh Tutankhamun, who died in 1323 B.C.

Celery should be on anyone's shopping list!

ASK DR. LIZ #9

ARE YOU CHICKEN?

Q: Is it true that eating chicken today can be a health hazard?
A: Yes, sadly there can be a very high cost to cheap chicken! Consumer reports published a study in February 2014 finding 97 percent of retail chicken breast from grocery store shelves was contaminated with bacteria that can make people sick.[11]

Q: Why is that?
A: Consumer reports suggests that the cramped conditions on factory chicken farms may play a role. New research indeed shows overcrowding can increase salmonella invasion and fecal contamination.

Q: Is poultry the cause of most outbreaks of salmonella?
A: Yes! Salmonella found in poultry, particularly chicken, is the leading cause of food poisoning, food poisoning hospitalization, and is the number one food poisoning related death.

Q: Isn't it illegal to sell poultry contaminated with dangerous bacteria?
A: Sadly, it can be deadly, but not illegal. Every year in America, over 200,000 people get salmonella poisoning! Due to strengthening of food safety regulation under the Clinton Administration, this has decreased from 390,000 people per year to 200,000. This is still too many people getting unnecessarily sick, primarily from eating chicken, don't you think so?

Q: Why do so many people die from salmonella?
A: One of the most concerning developments in medicine is the emergence of bacterial super resistance to multiple classes of drugs. More than ¼ of chicken salmonella cases are resistant to not one, but five different treatment drugs.

Q: Is all chicken equal?
A: Organic chicken is definitely better than conventional chicken, but is still found to be contaminated in 84 percent of the cases.

Q: How can that be? I thought organic chicken was safe?
A: Organic chickens are still slaughtered typically in the same factory farms. You know what I'm going to say: a plant-based diet is best and safest.

I am chicken to eat chicken!

ASK DR. LIZ #10

BENEFITS OF COCONUT OIL

ANTI-AGING

o Pure virgin coconut oil is found to have many dermatological benefits including anti-aging
o Moisturizes and beautifies the skin
o Eliminates wrinkles
o Promotes the production of collagen

HEART HEALTH

o Clears blockages in the arteries and promotes heart health
o Helps raise the good HDL (high density lipoproteins) cholesterol, which in turn helps lower bad LDL (low density lipoproteins) cholesterol
o Other oils, such as vegetable oil, clogs arteries
o Cooking oils like canola, corn, soy, safflower, and sunflower are loaded with omega-6 fats, which cause heart disease and do many other bad things to the body

SKIN HEALTH

o Good for the skin
o Put on insect bites, bruises, sunburns

IMMUNITY

o Although coconut oil is a saturated fat, it does have lauric acid, which strengthens your body's ability to fight off bacteria and viruses effectively. Pure virgin refined coconut oil is considered by many research scientists to be the healthiest oil in the world!

ASK DR. LIZ #11

TELL ME ABOUT DEPRESSION

Q: Can you tell me about depression?
A: Depression can be defined as feelings of severe despondency and dejection. Despondency is a state of low spirits caused by loss of hope or loss of courage. Dejection is being in a sad state. Depression is when an individual feels sad and has lost hope.

Q: What kind of symptoms does someone with depression experience?
A: Depression can cause severe symptoms that affect how you feel, think, and handle daily activities, such as sleeping, eating and working. To be diagnosed with depression, the symptoms must be present for at least two weeks. Some of the signs and symptoms of depression include:

- A persistent sad or anxious mood
- Feelings of hopelessness or pessimism
- Irritability
- Feelings of guilt, worthlessness, or helplessness
- Loss of interest or pleasure in hobbies and activities
- Decreased energy or fatigue
- Moving or talking more slowly
- Feeling restless or having trouble sitting still
- Difficulty concentrating, remembering, or making decisions
- Difficulty sleeping, early morning awakening, or oversleeping
- Appetite and or weight changes
- Thoughts of death or suicide, or suicide attempts
- Aches or pains, headaches, cramps, or digestive problems without a clear physical cause and/or that do not ease even with treatment
- Not everyone who is depressed experiences every symptom. Some people experience only a few, whereas others may experience many.
- Several persistent symptoms in addition to low mood are required for a diagnosis major depression.

Q: Are there different types of depression?
A: Yes. Some forms of depression are slightly different:

1. In persistent depressive disorder, also called dysthymia, the person must have episodes of major depression along with periods of less severe symptoms, but symptoms must last for two years to be considered persistent depressive disorder.

2. Perinatal depression is another form of depression that women can experience after child delivery and is much more serious than the *baby blues*. This can occur during pregnancy or post pregnancy.
3. Psychotic depression occurs when a person has severe depression plus some form of psychosis, such as having disturbing false fixed beliefs, delusions, or hearing or seeing upsetting things that others cannot hear or see (hallucinations). The psychotic symptoms typically have a depressive theme such as delusions of guilt, poverty, or illness.
4. Seasonal affective disorder is characterized by the onset of depression during the winter months when there is less sunlight. This depression generally lifts during the spring and summer. Winter depression is typically accompanied by social withdrawal, increased sleep, and weight gain, and predictably returns every year in seasonal affective disorder.

Q: What about bipolar disorder?
A: Bipolar disorder is different from depression. A person with bipolar disorder experiences episodes of extremely low moods that meet the criteria for major depression, but the person with bipolar disorder also experiences extreme high-euphoric or irritable moods called *mania* or a less severe form called *hypomania*.

Q: Are there other types of depressive disorders?
A: Newly added to the diagnostic classification for depressive disorders includes disruptive mood dysregulation disorder (diagnosed in children and adolescents). This condition has extreme irritability, anger, and frequent, intense temper outbursts. Premenstrual dysphoric disorder (a.k.a. PMDD) is a severe form of premenstrual syndrome (PMS) and follows a predictable cyclic pattern. Symptoms begin in the late luteal phase of the menstrual cycle, after ovulation and before menstruation.

Q: Is it common for people to experience depression?
A: Yes, depression is a common serious mood disorder according to the National Institute of Mental Health.

Q: Who mainly experiences depression?
A: One in ten Americans suffer from depression. One depression fact that holds true across racial and economic differences is that depression is twice as common in women than it is in men. Major depression is most likely to affect people between the ages of forty-five and sixty-five. People in the middle age are at the top of the bell curve for depression, but the people at each end of the curve, the very young and the very old, may be at higher risk for severe depression. In fact, late life depression affects about six million Americans, but 90 percent of them never seek help.

Q: Does the geriatric population suffer from severe depression and risk of suicide?
A: At some level yes! Studies show that older Americans who are severely depressed and have thoughts of suicide are sadly, but more likely to succeed at committing suicide. When a young person attempts suicide, they are not as sure and are often revived from their attempt. Whereas when a senior attempts a suicide, they much more commonly succeed at doing so.

Q: What can we do to support our elder population in general to ensure feelings of love?
A: Our elder population needs and deserves to feel loved and needed. That's what each and every one of us can do for elders in our own family, in our community, at our churches, etc. It is important to reach out, touch, and hug an elder person. Oftentimes, the elderly don't get to experience love through touch and this, in itself, is vital for the elderly.

Q: Do many people take antidepressants?
A: Over 13 percent of Americans report taking antidepressants, according to a 2018 report from the National Center of Health Statistics.

Q: What exactly are antidepressants?
A: Antidepressants are drugs that act on specific brain chemicals which regulate your mood. Antidepressant take time (usually two to four weeks) to work. Antidepressants are the second most commonly prescribed medication in the United States, according to the American Psychological Association. The first being analgesics, which are drugs prescribed to treat pain.

Q: Would you speak to us about the types of antidepressants?
A: Yes, of course. There are many different types of drugs used to treat depression including SSRIs, SNRIs, NDRIs, tricyclics and MAOIs to name a few.

Q: What is the most common type of antidepressants?
A: I bet you've heard of Prozac. It is an example of an SSRI, which stands for selective serotonin reuptake inhibitor. Prozac and Zoloft are examples of an SSRI. SSRIs work by increasing levels of serotonin in the brain. They block the reabsorption of serotonin in the brain, making more serotonin available.

An SNRI example would be Cymbalta. SNRI involves Norepinephrine, and is related to alertness and energy. SNRIs block both serotonin and norepinephrine from going back into the cells that released them.

Wellbutrin is an example of an NDRI. NDRIs involve dopamine and norepinephrine, and work similarly to SSRIs. These are fairly common ones.

Tricyclics and MAOIs are not any longer commonly used due to the potential dangers they cause to patients, which include side effects and interactions with other medications.

Q: Do antidepressants even work?
A: Studies show that pertaining to mild to moderate depression, they work, but only as effectively as a placebo, and placebos do work. For someone with an extreme condition of depression, antidepressants are found to be effective.

Q: What can someone do if they don't want to take an antidepressant and they suffer from mild to moderate depression?
A: Exercise and eat an anti-inflammatory diet. It's this simple. If depression can be induced with pro-inflammatory drugs, might an anti-inflammatory diet be effective in preventing and treating

mood disorders? People who are depressed have higher levels of CRP, or C-reactive proteins markers in their blood.

Q: What are the diets of most people that are depressed?
A: People who eat more soda and refined meat have greater tendencies toward depressions. Omega-3s don't help with depression or anti-inflammation.

Q: What kinds of foods should I consume if I am depressed?
A: It is key to consume antioxidant rich foods which include fresh, organic fruits and vegetables, and folate rich beans and greens. It is important that antioxidants are consumed thorough food not supplements, it is shown that people suffering from depression and mood disorders can and do improve with an anti-inflammatory plant-based diet of antioxidant rich foods.

Q: Can I eat fish?
A: No, I don't recommend eating fish for depression.

Q: Why is that?
A: The mercury content in fish may help explain links found between fish intake and mental disorders, depression, and suicide.

Q: Can you provide me with a summary?
A: Studies show that if you suffer from mild to moderate depression, you are better off to exercise and eat an anti-inflammatory diet than to take an antidepressant drug therapy, which only works as effectively as a placebo.

ASK DR. LIZ #12

DIABETES

Q: What causes type 2 diabetes?
A: Saturated fat can be a major contributor to the onset of type 2 diabetes.

Q: What is it about saturated fat that can do this?
A: When there is too much saturated fat in the human body, it can be toxic to the beta cells in the pancreas. The beta cells in the pancreas are the cells that produce insulin; thus, they can debilitate insulin secretion. After our teen years, our body has all of the insulin producing beta cells we will ever have. It is shown that saturated fat is the key contributor to beta cell death. Diets full in saturated fat are the most toxic to these beta cells.

Q: So, we must not consume saturated fats in order to avoid type 2 diabetes?
A: Absolutely! Like smoking, not all people who do smoke die of lung cancer or even get lung cancer, but obviously, their risk is increased. The same is true for saturated fat and diabetes.

Q: How can we prevent getting diabetes?
A: Studies show those who eat the most legumes are less likely to develop diabetes. Those who ate at least three servings of beans weekly were much less likely to develop metabolic syndrome or diabetes. These same people had lower body weight and a smaller waistline, too. Reducing belly fat may be the most effective way in treating Diabetes. Reducing body weight by creating nutritional ketosis is extremely helpful in preventing, managing, and eliminating type 2 diabetes.[13]

Be inspired to eat healthier, lose weight, and eat more legumes!

ASK DR. LIZ #13

ENERGY DENSITY

Q: What is energy density?
A: Energy density is a relatively new concept that is an important factor in body weight. It is defined as the amount of energy (calories) per unit weight of a food or beverage. For example, water provides a significant amount of weight without adding calories; fiber does, too. Foods high in water or fiber are generally lower in energy density. Whereas foods high in fat are high in energy density. This is because dietary fat provides the greatest amount of energy per gram (calories per unit weight).

Q: What are some high energy density foods?
A: The CDC offers some examples such as bacon, which has many calories in a small package. A bagel is an example of a medium energy density food. Low energy density foods are typified as fruits and vegetables. The lower the energy density of the food, the better.

Q: Are there any exceptions?
A: There are two exceptions. Nuts have so much fat that they appear less healthy than they are. Soda, on the other hand, appears less harmful than it actually is. Otherwise, the "science" supports a relationship between energy density and body weight. Consuming diets lower in energy density may be an effective strategy for managing body weight.

Q: Why is that?
A: People tend to eat a consistent weight of food. So, when there are fewer calories per pound, caloric intake is reduced. Energy density can be reduced in a variety of ways, such as the addition of fruits and vegetables, by lowering fat content, or by lowering sugar content.

Q: Do you feel full on fewer calories when you eat a diet full of low density foods?
A: Yes. Many organizations apply this framework to their highly successful diet plans including the mayo clinic, the National Institute of Health, and the CDC to name a few. Ideally, one must look at three areas of lifestyle that may require change such as food, exercise and sleep in order to make weight loss sustainable.

Q: How does sleep impact weight loss?
A: Sleep is important for weight loss. Most adults require eight hours of sleep. The less sleep you get, the higher your weight tends to be. Sleep impacts hunger and satiety hormones. Getting enough sleep is a lifestyle factor that is essential to successful weight loss.

ASK DR. LIZ #14

FERTILITY: TIPS FOR GETTING PREGNANT

Q: I want to have a baby, but I'm having difficulty getting pregnant. What is something I can try?
A: One of the best ways to become pregnant, is to do so through the use of Traditional Chinese Medicine. By using acupuncture and sometimes herbs, many people are able to conceive a child who otherwise have been unsuccessful doing so. Better yet, it is often fast and cost-effective.

Q: How does it work?
A: It's incredible how effective acupuncture alone works for fertility success! Whether the woman is experiencing irregular menstruation or the male has a lower than optimal sperm count, acupuncture can help both scenarios. Acupuncture is not only shown to effectively regulate menstruation, it can also boost male sperm count by over one million in a single visit!

Q: How many visits are required to get long-term sustainable results?
A: We normally get results for a pregnancy in less than six months, normally within ninety days! Depending on the situation, we work with the couple to create what they most desire – a happy, healthy family.

Q: What happens if I have PCOS, endometriosis, or fibroid tumors?
A: We have excellent success in many cases. It's best for you to come in for an evaluation.

Q: What about IVF, in vitro fertilization?
A: Some of our patients will use both modalities to become pregnant – in vitro fertilization and acupuncture treatments. Others just come for acupuncture and herbals. Acupuncture greatly increases the odds of fertility success. We often get results in half the time, at half the price.

Q: Are there specific types of foods to Increase Fertility?
A: Fresh fruits and vegetables, along with red organic grass-fed beef. Beef is rich in iron. Oftentimes, women are blood deficient, or slightly anemic, which makes it more difficult to conceive and then hold the baby. To optimize the ability to conceive a healthy child and then carry the fetus full-term, one of the things we do is ensure they have a good amount of red blood cell count (RBC) and hemoglobin.

Q: Are there other foods you recommend for a healthy pregnancy?
A: I encourage women to eat figs, berries, particularly strawberries, beans, sweet potato, and seaweed. Stay away from alcohol and sugar.

ASK DR. LIZ #15

FOLK REMEDY VS. TCM

Q: Tell us about TCM?
A: TCM is an abbreviation for Traditional Chinese Medicine. TCM is a growing healthcare practice in the United States and around the world. It is used to help people heal from many diseases. The World Health Organization has now mandated that best practices of medicine must include both biomedicine and TCM.

Q: What does TCM practice include?
A: TCM practice includes the use of many modalities of healing including but not limited to acupuncture, physical therapy (Tui Na), custom therapeutics, herbal remedies, gua sha, cupping, medical Qigong, and more. To become a TCM doctor or practitioner in the United States, one must be boarded in acupuncture, herbology, foundational Chinese medicine and Western medicine.

Q: Is a doctor of acupuncture and oriental medicine the same as an acupuncturist?
A: A DAOM is a higher level than a basic acupuncturist who has obtained a master's degree. A TCM doctor has a higher level of training. A DAOM typically attends school for ten to eleven years. This includes four years of undergraduate college, four years of medical school, and two to four years of post-medical school specialty training (similar to standard medical school).

Q: What is the difference between folk remedy and TCM herbs?
A: Folk remedy often uses one herb or one food to treat an ailment. In TCM, custom formulas are mixed to effectively treat the condition.

Q: Can you give an example?
A: Say a patient has pneumonia. An example of a folk remedy would be to boil red onions, limes, and add honey, cool slightly, then drink. Whereas TCM would offer a variety of thirty-four different base formulas varying from Chai Hu Gui Zhi Gan Jiang Tang that can treat anything from bronchitis, pneumonia, influenza, hepatitis, cholecystitis to the common cold to Wei Jing Tang that will treat asthmatic issues, pertussis and pneumonia. How do you know which one? TCM takes into consideration the individual's constitution.

Q: What is a constitution?
A: A constitution is an individual's nature. An example would be that some people run "hot" versus "cold," meaning some people tend to feel warm more, they prefer cold water to drink, or others may have cold limbs. Different constitutions require different treatment. With pneumonia, each individual would need to be treated uniquely to achieve effective results to resolve the pneumonia due to the difference in constitutions.

Q: TCM can be a very effective personalized solution to healthcare. Would you give us one more example of folk remedy versus TCM?

A: Yes. Turmeric is a well-known and effective herb than can be used relatively safely. It's an anti-inflammatory and can help treat pain above the umbilicus. If you also have pain in your legs, you must consider an additional strategy for effectiveness. TCM is all-encompassing and does this.

ASK DR. LIZ #16

GUT HEALTH

Q: What is gut health?
A: Gut health mainly pertains to digestion and the pH balance in the body. Strong emotional feelings can trigger digestive issues ranging from Crohn's disease, irritable bowel syndrome, leaky gut to stomach ulcer or pancreatitis. "A healthy garden needs healthy soil." The soil is our flora, which is found throughout the body, largely in the intestines of the digestive system.

Q: Why is gut health so important?
A: Gut health is so very important to a well-functioning human body. A healthy gut provides protection to us from infection and disease. If you go back to the most ancient medical literature, it has been stated that "the body center" is the true function of our, what we call today, the "immune system."

Q: What makes a gut healthy?
A: A healthy "gut" depends upon the health of the digestive organs which include the mouth, the stomach, the intestines–both the small and large–along with the liver, gallbladder, spleen, and pancreas.

Q: Can you tell us about the flora in our gut?
A: Interestingly, nobody really knows what the correct balance or correct amount of flora should be here in the United States. This is because there has been such wide usage of antibiotics, which are known to destroy much of the good flora in the body. One solution is to take a good probiotic. Garden of Life RAW has over 85 billion, offering a large and diverse bunch of varied good bacteria. They make probiotics for women, women over fifty, men, men over fifty, etc.

Q: What are some foods that can help promote gut health?
A: Kombucha.

Q: Tell me more about the gut, Liz.
A: The gut was often considered the second brain. You know when we say to each other, "I have a 'gut' feeling"? Well, there is a reason for that. The dopamine and serotonin in the gut actually send messages to the brain to protect us, if the gut is healthy.

Q: Can a healthy gut help protect us from different diseases?
A: Yes. A healthy gut can help protect us from a wide range of diseases including depression, rheumatoid arthritis, chronic fatigue, and more.

ASK DR. LIZ #17

HEART HEALTH AND CARDIOVASCULAR DISEASE

Q: Tell us about our heart?
A: As you know, our heart is very important. Heart health can refer to any kind of cardiovascular disease, not only the "heart" organ itself. In fact, cardiovascular disease is the number one killer in America, but it doesn't have to be. I will give you some tips today on how not to die from cardiovascular disease. In oriental medicine, the heart is known as the "emperor" and is considered to be the most important visceral organ. It is more important than the brain because it houses the mind. The heart is in charge of the vessels, so we want to not only make our "emperor" strong and healthy, we want our "vessels" to be strong and healthy, too! Our vessels would be our arteries, veins, and capillaries.

Q: So how does that work?
A: All of our organs, veins, arteries, and capillaries are lined with what is called "endothelium." If the endothelium is clogged with plaque, then the capillaries, veins, and arteries are also clogged. Our capillaries, veins, and arteries are the pathways where blood and oxygen is carried and transported throughout our bodies. So, if the pathways are clogged, blood and oxygen cannot get through to nourish our body and ischemia, a heart attack or a stroke occurs. This build of plaque on our endothelium is known as atherosclerosis. Sadly, most Americans raised on a conventional diet have significant plaque accumulation inside the coronary arteries, and this is why heart disease is our number one killer![14]

Q: What is the plaque made up of?
A: Plaque is made up of fat, calcium and other substances found in the blood. Over time, plaque hardens inside of your arteries and narrows your coronary arteries. This limits the oxygen rich blood to the heart.

Q: What is endothelium?
A: Endothelium is actually skin that lines all of our organs and vessels, including all our arteries, capillaries, and veins. So, we not only have skin on the outside of our bodies, we have it on the inside of our bodies, too.

Q: Is that what happens when someone gets a heart attack or a stroke?
A: Most commonly, yes.

Q: What is the best thing to reduce risk of cardiovascular disease?
A: Stop smoking, get regular exercise, and change your diet. A gram of fiber daily from whole grains is associated with a lower chance of dying from a heart attack and reduces risk of cancer, diabetes, and respiratory diseases as well as lowers the risk of dying from infection.[14] It's best to consume a traditional Mediterranean diet.

Q: What does a Mediterranean diet consist of?
A: It includes whole grains, fruits, vegetables, lentils, beans, nuts, and seeds.

Q: What if someone wants to take care of their heart health, but is gluten intolerant? What types of "whole grains" should they eat?
A: Whole grains that are gluten free and help protect your heart include quinoa and teff, which is the staple grain of Ethiopia and one of the smallest grains in the world. Teff is a good source of iron, calcium, protein, fiber, and B vitamins. Sorghum is highly nutritious and cost-effective gluten free grain, also high in the B vitamins as well as in magnesium, iron, calcium, copper, potassium, and protein. Buckwheat, despite its name, is not a form of wheat. It lowers cholesterol and blood pressure levels, is high in antioxidants, is shown to help prevent the onset of type 2 diabetes, and has a variety of vitamins and minerals. You can also incorporate a variety of rice.

Q: What if someone is a vegan or a vegetarian? Can their diet protect heart health?
A: Vegetarian or vegan diets may also work, too, but it must be accompanied by vitamin B12. Most likely because of the anti-inflammatory effects from fiber.

Q: How many people die each year from heart disease?
A: About 610,000 people die of heart disease in the United States every year. That's one in four deaths. Heart disease is the leading cause of death for both men and women. Strokes kill about 5 million people each year worldwide and is the top neurological disorder that debilitates people.

Q: Should we all take aspirin to prevent heart disease?
A: The benefits of taking a daily aspirin must be weighed against the risk of internal bleeding.

Q: Is there a natural form of aspirin?
A: Yes. Salicylic acid, the active ingredient in aspirin, has been used for thousands of years as an anti-inflammatory and pain killer in the form of willow tree bark extract. Hippocrates originally used this to treat fever and alleviate pain during child birth. It also acts as a blood thinner. For those who have already had a heart attack, the benefits are clear that taking a low dosage of aspirin daily is a good thing to do; however, for those who have not had a previous issue, the studies show differently.

Q: Are there any scientific methods to elongate life through cardiovascular practice?
A: Interestingly, the number of heartbeats per lifetime is remarkably similar, whether you are a hamster, whale, or human. If humans are predetermined to approximately 3 billion heart rates per lifetime, can slowing the cardiovascular system increase life span?

Q: How do we put our fingers on the pulse of longevity?
A: To maximize lifespan, the target resting heart rate may be one beat per second or less.

Q: Do people with slower hearts live longer?
A: Yes. A fast heart rate may lead to a higher death rate, leading to heart disease or heart failure. This information is independent of the level of physical activity. A fast heart rate is not only a marker of risk, but a bona fide risk factor. This information is now well-recognized. Lowering a heart rate

lowers our death rate. This has been shown in at least eight clinical trials. One beat per second is the optimal goal.

Q: Is there any secret in medicine?
A: The best kept secret in medicine, is under the right conditions, the body heals itself.
Heart disease is reversible! Originally, researchers blamed the animal fat or animal protein, but attention has recently shifted to bacterial toxins known as "endotoxins." Certain foods such as meats harbor bacteria that trigger inflammation. In Dr. Ornish's studies, Dr. Ornish reported a 91 percent reduction in angina attacks within just a few weeks in patients placed on a plant-based diet, with or without exercise.

Q: So, animal saturated fat is not actually the real culprit?
A: No. It is the endotoxins that are more concerning to the research scientists than the fat itself, according to recent clinical findings. Pork, poultry, and dairy along with other animal products show endotoxins causing inflammation within an hour after eating. The cause? Coming from the food itself.

Q: What is an endotoxin?
A: An endotoxin is a form of sugar and is associated with gram-negative bacteria. The impact of endotoxins in the human body includes diseases such as E. coli, meningitis, bordetella, and cholera to name a few diseases that stem from gram negative bacteria.

Q: Can we eat fish? Do they have endotoxins?
A: According to the National Institute of Health, compared to mammals, fish are resistant to endotoxic shock. Therefore, endotoxins are not found to be an issue in our seafood.

Q: Can you talk to us about cholesterol and the impact that it has on heart health?
A: Sure. The first thing to understand about cholesterol, is that it is NOT a fat. Cholesterol is a hormone. Triglycerides are fats, cholesterol is not. Cholesterol is needed to make hormones, vitamin D, and substances that help with digestion. People are way overmedicated with cholesterol medications, and inappropriately so in many cases. The ratio is what is most important when it comes to heart health. To calculate your cholesterol ratio, divide your high-density-lipoprotein (HDL or good cholesterol) number into your total cholesterol number. An optimal ratio is 3.5 or less.

Q: What is considered a desirable level of cholesterol?
A: A desirable level of total cholesterol for adults without heart disease is less than 200 mg/dL. An HDL cholesterol level of 60 mg/dL and above is considered protective against heart disease, while a level of less than 50 mg/dL or 40mg/dL for men is considered a major risk factor for heart disease. A low LDL cholesterol is best to prevent heart attack or stroke. Lower than 100 mg/dL is the ideal. So, if your total cholesterol is 200 and your HDL is 60, your ratio is 3.33 which is good, because it's less than 3.5. On the other hand, if your total cholesterol is 300 and your HDL is 100, there is nothing wrong with that either. However, if you have 180 total cholesterol and only a 40 HDL, your ratio is 4.5 which is not so good. So, as you can see, ratio is more important than total cholesterol levels when it comes to heart health.

Q: What about hypertension? Can you tell us about that?
A: Hypertension is another name for high blood pressure. It measures the force of the blood against your artery walls. Blood pressure is determined by both by the amount of blood your heart pumps and the amount of resistance to blood flow in your arteries. The more blood your heart pumps and the narrower your arteries, the higher your blood pressure.

Q: Can you have high blood pressure without knowing it?
A: You sure can, so it's a good idea to monitor your blood pressure.

Q: How can you lower blood pressure?
A: Eat a healthy Mediterranean style diet, limit white breads, limit alcohol, limit sodium, and limit sugar. Exercise regularly and lose weight. When you lose extra pounds, your blood pressure will drop.

Q: What should our blood pressure be?
A: Normal blood pressure according to the American Heart Association is no more than 120/80. Systolic is less than 120 and Diastolic is less than 80. Prehypertension is 120-140 and diastolic 80-90. High blood pressure stage 1 is 140-160/90-100, stage 2 is 160 or higher/100 or higher, and hypertensive crisis is 180/110 or higher.

Q: Give us some tips, Liz?
A: Here are a few key tips based to help you live longer and prevent and or reverse heart disease:

1. Eat fresh fruits and vegetables, preferably organic and cleaned (lowers inflammation)
2. Eat Brazil nuts (lowers cholesterol). Brazil nuts bring down LDL 'bad' cholesterol faster than statin drugs, so eat those if you have high cholesterol.
3. Use organic coconut oil (lowers LDL)
4. Meditate (improves heart health by calming the mind). Practice this each morning and before you go to bed. Mind clearing helps your heart health.
5. Move, walk, do yoga, Tai Chi, Chi Gong, bicycle, swim… (helps restore endothelium)
6. Prepare your food so it is not cold, including your fruits and vegetables (facilitates digestion)
7. Incorporate these five spices into your diet: garlic (antibiotic), ginger (aids digestion), turmeric (lessens inflammation), cayenne pepper (stimulates circulation) and onions (cleans blood)
8. Green tea (lowers LDL and triglycerides)
9. Harmonize your relationships, work environment, and your home (improves heart health by lessening stress and mind calming)

If you want additional information I highly recommend Michael Greger, M.D.'s book, *How Not to Die*.

Q: Why did you choose to give us nine tips?
A: Nine is a symbol of infinity, immortality, or everlasting. So, since our goal is to live long healthy lives, I thought nine was appropriate.

Q: What would an oriental medical doctor suggest to someone with a 'weak' heart?

A: In addition to many of these tips, a doctor of oriental medicine would also suggest, eat hearts! Yes, you read correctly. If you have a weak heart, eat hearts! You can find chicken hearts in your local supermarket, and beef hearts you may need to shop around for. Interesting, but true. How to eat them? You can sauté them in a little bit of coconut oil in a frying pan. Really amazing!

ASK DR. LIZ #18

FOODS FOR HEART HEALTH

Q: Would you share with me what you believe to be the best foods for a healthy heart?
A: I would have to include flaxseed, blueberries, oatmeal, salmon, green tea, and legumes. Heart disease is the leading cause of death for people in the United States, so let's eat healthier to change these statistics!

1. Flaxseed is known to reverse heart disease and help prevent cancer, stroke, and diabetes. Interesting history of flax seed is that flax seed was cultivated in Babylon as early as 3000 B.C. King Charlemagne created laws that mandated people consume it because he believed so strongly in the health benefits of it! Now, thirteen centuries later, some call it the most powerful plant food on the planet!
2. Blueberries help to lower blood pressure!
3. Oatmeal lowers cholesterol! It is best to avoid instant oatmeal because it does not have the full effect. If you are gluten intolerant, I recommend Bob's Red Mill steel cut oats because it is gluten free and wheat free!
4. Salmon helps to regulate heartbeat and reduce plaque buildup. It is best to eat twice a week.
5. Green tea improves blood vessel function within thirty minutes after consumption. Drink green tea daily to improve the health of your arteries.
6. Legumes like peas, lentils, and beans can substantially strengthen your heart health by nearly 25 percent and help control blood sugar if eaten four to five times a week.

Q: How do I use flax seed in my everyday living?
A: The flaxseed must be ground, and you can buy it this way. Just take 1 teaspoon to 1 tablespoon a day by sprinkling it on cereal or by putting it into a smoothie. Flaxseed also promotes healthy digestion, regulates bowel movements, promotes breast and brain health, and helps balance hormones! Yes, you strike gold when you decide to take flaxseed!

Q: Are other berries good for heart health as well?
A: Yes! Other berries are also good for heart health. They have high levels of vitamin C, fiber, and antioxidants. It's not only blueberries that are good for your health; however, they are known specifically for protecting your heart. Blueberries lower blood pressure, improve blood flow, and reduce risk of heart attack, so enjoy your daily dose!

Q. What about goji berries?
A. Goji berries are delicious and extremely healthy!

Q: Are goji berries good for my heart?
A: Yes! They will help lessen or remove heart palpitations, improve your energy level, lessen anxiety, and help with insomnia. They are also very good for the kidney!

ASK DR. LIZ #19

HI, HONEY!

Q: Is honey good for me?
A: Yes! Honey is very good for you!

Q: What does it do for me?
A: Honey contains antioxidants and enzymes that have healthy effects on the body.

Q: Does honey help me to lose weight?
A: Yes! If you combine honey with cinnamon, it can help to accelerate weight loss if used in conjunction with an otherwise healthy diet.

<u>Recipe</u>
1 cup hot water
½ teaspoon cinnamon
1 teaspoon raw organic honey

<u>Instructions</u>
Drink first thing in the morning. Mix cinnamon with hot water and let it cool.
Add honey. Wait half an hour before eating.

Q: What is manuka honey?
A: It is a honey from New Zealand that has an amazing nutritional value.

Q: What makes it so special?
A: Manuka honey has up to four times the amount of nutrition of regular honey and has a considerably higher number of live enzymes. It contains amino acids, B vitamins, calcium, iron, magnesium, manganese, potassium, and zinc.

Q: What type of Manuka honey do I need?
A: Manuka honey is marketed for use in many conditions including:
- Preventing or treating cancer
- Reducing high cholesterol
- Reducing systemic inflammation
- Treating diabetes
- Treating eye, ear, and sinus infections
- Treating gastrointestinal problems
- Treating wounds and leg ulcers
- Preventing gingivitis and periodontal disease
- Reduction of inflammation of the esophagus

Q: Can I use honey to look better?
A: Yes! Any kind of honey helps the skin become moist or keeps the skin moist. You can spread 1 tablespoon of raw honey on clean dry skin and let it sit for twenty minutes. Rinse with tepid water. Honey can also help fade scars, treat acne, hydrate the body, moisturize cuticles, relieve sunburn, and condition and add shine to the hair!

All I can say is, "Hi, honey, I'm home!"

ASK DR. LIZ #20

KIDNEY DISEASE

Q: Tell us about our kidneys?
A: Our kidneys remove waste products from our blood and regulate our water metabolism.

Q: So, our kidneys are a filtration system?
A: Yes. Our kidneys are responsible for filtering the bad stuff from our blood and eliminating that bad stuff out of our bodies through our urine.

Q: What is kidney failure?
A: Kidney failure refers to the loss of function of our kidneys' ability to eliminate waste and regulate water levels in our body. Interestingly, we can live with kidney disease without even knowing it for a long time. Within our kidneys, we have nephrons, which are essential in the filtration process of cleaning our blood and keeping our bodies healthy. We have approximately 2.5 million nephrons in our kidneys. Interestingly, you can function normally with only 30 percent of those nephrons working.

Q: So, you could have severe kidney damage with no symptoms?
A: Yes. We can function normally without experiencing symptoms when 70 percent of our nephrons within our kidney are not functioning before we would experience any symptoms, or very few. In advanced stages of kidney disease, dangerous levels of wastes and fluids back up in your body.

Q: What are some of the symptoms of kidney failure?
A: According to the American Kidney Fund, symptoms may include itching, muscle cramps, nausea and vomiting, loss of appetite, selling in the feet, change in urination (either more or less), trouble catching your breath, and difficulty sleeping. Blood pressure is also controlled by the kidneys.

Q: Can we prevent and treat kidney disease?
A: Kidney failure may be both prevented and treated with a plant-based diet, and no wonder! Kidneys are highly vascular organs. Harvard researchers found three significant dietary risk factors for kidney decline in function: animal protein, animal fat, and cholesterol. Animal fat can alter the actual structure of our kidneys by clogging up the human kidneys shown in autopsies. Animal protein can have a profound effect on normal kidney function, what's called hyperfiltration, causing an increase workload of the kidney, and watch an increase pressure in the kidneys, but not plant protein. Plant protein does not have this effect.

Q: Is it okay to eat plant protein?
A: Yes. Eggs, meat, and dairy create high levels of acid which lead to tubular toxicity in our kidneys.

Q: How does fish, pork, or poultry affect the kidneys?

A: Fish, pork, and poultry are the worst! Eat a meal of tuna fish, and you can see the increased pressure on the kidneys go up one to three hours after the meal in both non-diabetics and diabetics. So, we are not talking about the effects decades down the road, but just hours after it goes into our mouth.

Q: What about vegetable protein?
A: If instead of having a tuna fish salad sandwich you had a tofu salad sandwich that has the exact same amount of protein, what happens? No effect. There is no problem.

Q: Why does animal protein cause this overload reaction, but not plant protein?
A: It appears to be due to the inflammation triggered by the consumption of animal products.

Q: How do we know that?
A: Because if you give a powerful anti-inflammatory drug along with that tuna fish, you can abolish that hyperfiltration protein leakage response to meat ingestion. Then there is the acid load. Animal foods, meat, eggs, and dairy induce the formation of acid within the kidneys which may lead to tubular toxicity damage within the kidneys. Animal foods tend to be acid forming, especially fish, which is the worst, and pork and poultry. Whereas plant food tends to be relatively neutral or alkaline, base forming to counteract the acid, so the key to halting the progression of chronic kidney disease might be in the produce market, rather than the pharmacy.

Q: Have plant-based diets been used to treat kidney disease?
A: Yes, and no wonder plant-based diets have been used to treat kidney disease for decades. It can be clearly seen that by switching a patient on and off from a plant-based diet to conventional based diet the kidney function goes up and down like a light switch based on what goes into their mouths. [14]

ASK DR. LIZ #21

DIET FOR KIDNEY HEALTH

Q: Who is most prone to kidney disease?
A: African Americans, Hispanics, and American Indians are at high risk for developing kidney failure. This is due in part to high rates of diabetes and high blood pressure in these communities.

Q: Do plant-based diets protect against kidney cancer?
A: Yes. Plant-based diets appear to protect against renal cell carcinoma both directly and indirectly.

Q: Do lots of people get kidney cancer?
A: Over 58,000 Americans are diagnosed with kidney cancer every year and 13,000 die.

Q: What seems to be the cause?
A: Nitrates from animal products and sodium intake.

Q: Don't vegetables also have nitrates in them?
A: Some do; however, they do not produce the same negative impact on health.

Q: What specifically is known to help reverse kidney failure?
A: The Kempner rice diet.

Q: What is the Kempner rice diet?
A: Walter Kempner, a physician scientist from Duke University, created the Kempner rice-fruit diet. He found that a low protein diet helped with kidney function.

Q: How were the results?
A: Two-thirds of the patients on his rice-fruit diet had reversal of kidney failure. People had just a few months to live and then they got better in a matter of five months.

Q: Has this been documented in medical literature?
A: An editorial in New England Journal of Medicine described Kempner's results as just short of miraculous.

Q: What's in the Kempner rice diet?
A: Dry rice of 250-350 grams daily. The rice cannot contain any salt or milk product. The rice is boiled or steamed in water or fruit juice without salt or fat.

Q: Is anything else allowed?
A: Fruit and fruit juice are allowed. Dried fruits can be used as long as nothing but sugar has been added.

1 cup of dry rice = 200 grams
No avocadoes, dates, or nuts.
No tomato or vegetable juices. Supplemental vitamins are added:
vitamin A (5000 units), vitamin D (1000 units), thiamin chloride (5 mg), riboflavin (5 mg), niacin amide (25 mg), calcium pantothenate (2 mg). [14]

Q: How long does it take a patient to adapt to this diet?
A: Adaptation to the diet takes about two months. Exercise is encouraged. Bed rest is only advised with severe conditions. Water intake is restricted in some severely ill patients to less than six cups a day.

Thanks for sharing Walter's incredible findings!

ASK DR. LIZ #22

MUSHROOMS

Q: Are mushrooms good for me?
A: Yes. Mushrooms are high in vitamin D and iron. Consumption of mushrooms may lower our cholesterol. You may think twice about pushing them aside!

Q: Are mushrooms a vegetable?
A: No, all mushrooms are fungi.

Q: Which mushrooms fight cancer?
A: Shitake mushrooms fight tumors, both cancerous and non-cancerous tumors. Shitake is also very good for fighting infection. Maitake mushrooms are good for breast cancer. You can eat a half-cup a day to improve immune response. Reishi mushrooms are also good for anti-cancer effects, as well as anti-bacterial, anti-viral, and anti-fungal. Yes, you can fight fungus with fungus!

Q: Do mushrooms help protect us in other ways?
A: Studies show that consumption of mushrooms do also help with inflammation, particularly the porcini mushroom. The porcini mushroom is similar to the portabella mushroom.

Q: Can you tell me about the shimeji mushrooms?
A: Shimeji mushrooms are known to treat asthma, allergies, and diabetes.

Q: What about oyster mushrooms?
A: Oyster mushrooms are high in antioxidants and are being studied to treat HIV.

Q: What types of mushrooms do you like to eat?
A: I love all types of mushrooms. If you're a little hesitant to indulge in these little treasures, try getting a mixed package of white mushrooms and mix them in with a handful of shitake. Sautee them for seven plus minutes in coconut oil. Delicious!

ASK DR. LIZ #23

NUTRITIONAL YEAST

Helps to Prevent the Common Cold

Q: How is it best to prevent the common cold?
A: Interestingly, beta glucan fiber found in nutritional yeast, may improve immune function. We have been looking for centuries for natural immune modulators that will help regulate the immune system, all the while they have been sitting in the produce isle. Plants produce thousands of active compounds that help our bodies stay healthy, and certain types of fungi can help us boost immune function, too. Mushrooms, which are a form of fungi, have been used for many centuries to protect the body's defenses! An example would be, a type of fiber found in shitake mushrooms has been found to boost immune function! Shitake mushrooms are used in many countries such as Japan, China, and Eastern Russia as an "adjunct chemotherapy" and is injected intravenously in patients to fight cancers effectively.

Q: Tell me about beta glucan?
A: Beta glucan offers beneficial effects for the immune system and are found in bakers, brewers, and nutritional yeast.

Q: How do these beta glucans help our body when it comes to the common cold?
A: There have been over 6,000 papers written about beta glucans and their health benefits. A most recent study, double-blind placebo based, showed that by consuming just half to one teaspoon a day of nutritional yeast will reduce your chances of contracting the common cold by 25 percent.

Q: What precisely does it do to help me with sickness?
A: Beta glucans can help to maintain our bodies defense mechanism. People who took beta glucans were less likely to get sick with a cold, had fewer cold related sleeping difficulties, and less upper respiratory symptoms. Even mood was found to be improved! People that take beta glucans in this study described themselves as having increased "vigor"! The beta glucans counteract the negative effects of stress. They stimulate our immune defenses and they decrease inflammation by having an anti-inflammatory effect.

Q: What type and what brand will effectively build my immune system?
A: Braggs nutritional yeast is recommended because it has significantly less than a half a microgram of lead, which not only meets, but surpasses the California standard. For those of you folks who are unaware, California has higher standards for their food regulations than most states in the union to help protect people's health. Braggs meets the standard.[15]

ASK DR. LIZ #24

LET'S GO NUTS!

Q: Are Brazil nuts good for me?
A: Yes, a single serving of Brazil nuts may bring cholesterol levels of LDL and HDL down faster than statin drugs and keep cholesterol down even a month later after that single ingestion of just four nuts. Eat only four per month. More is NOT better.

Q: How long after you ingest the Brazil nuts does your cholesterol go down?
A: Just nine hours after eating the serving of four Brazil nuts, cholesterol went down an average of twenty points on the ten individuals in the study and stayed down for over thirty days. Statin drugs usually take four days.

Q: Which nuts best fight cancer?
A: Within hours, the blood of those fed walnuts were able to suppress the growth of breast cancer cells in a Petri dish study. Walnuts help to fight against cancer, not only breast cancer, but ALL cancers. This study was done at Penn State.

Q: Do walnuts help protect us in other ways?
A: Studies show that consumption of walnuts improve endothelium function along with healthy eating. Just eat about an ounce of walnuts a day.

Q: Which nuts might work best to fight cancer?
A: Walnuts and pecans took first place, with the bronze going to peanuts! Studies showed just eating two cups of nuts per week can help prevent pancreatic cancer.

Q: Which fruits work best to prevent cancer?
A: Cranberries and lemon took the title.

Q: What foods help to prevent against fibrocystic breast disease?
A: Featured data from the Harvard Nurses Study shows early nut consumption. Those eating more peanuts, nuts, beans, lentils, soybeans, or corn, including those folks with a family history, are less likely to develop breast cancer.[16]

ASK DR. LIZ #25

OXIDATIVE STRESS AND DIET

Q: Does what we eat really make a difference in our health?
A: Yes. Food is so important that it can actually prevent disease, and in many cases heal you from diseases that you don't want to get. Food actually has that much power to affect your body. The red blood cells in your body replace themselves entirely every 100 to 120 days. This continuous restorative process that the body goes through demands good nutrition in order to work properly. When the body isn't given enough fruits, vegetables, legumes, nuts, and spices, oxidative stress can cause the cells to break down, cause inflammation, and damage leading to cancer and chronic illness. These foods provide the body with antioxidants that destroy oxidative stress and keep the body healthy.

Q: What is oxidative stress?
A: Oxidative stress is essentially what happens when you slice an apple, leave it on the counter, and it turns brown. That is exactly what happens to our cells when we don't have enough antioxidants. Antioxidants destroy free radical activity, which is what causes oxidative stress. The key to the solution is to be sure to eat enough antioxidants, which are found in fruits and vegetables.

Q: If that is the case, why don't more doctors recommend foods to their patients?
A: More and more doctors incorporate healthy living, including nutrition, into their practice. But for doctors, this is also an education. They are not trained in medical school much on nutrition, but more so on cellular interaction with pharmaceuticals. Western medicine focuses on early detection vs. disease prevention and use mostly drugs and surgical procedures to solve problems. The powerful impact of good nutrition on disease prevention historically has not been well taught or studied in medical school here in the united states. Yet, good nutrition is key to quality living, disease prevention and longevity.

Q: When you say spices, what are you referring to?
A: There is a great article in this issue titled, "Four powerful spices that will help end disease." Be sure to read this one! This article talks about the power of garlic, turmeric, ginger and cayenne pepper, you will see each of these four spices have a concentrated power that help optimize your bodies performance. There are numerous studies showing that garlic kills cancer cells and herpes virus.

ASK DR. LIZ #26

HOW MUCH PROTEIN IS IDEAL AS WE AGE?

Q: What is the optimal amount of protein for senior citizens? Is there anything we can do to minimize muscle loss?
A: Yes. Interestingly protein is not a solution to maintaining muscle mass. The most effective solution to prevent muscle mass loss or to gain muscle mass is to eat vegetables and perform resistance training

Q: Why is that?
A: The alkalizing effects of vegetables may neutralize the mild metabolic acidosis in our body that facilitates the breakdown of muscle. Muscle wasting appears to be an adaptive response to acidosis. We all know when we exercise a muscle, it is likely to grow, or gain mass.

Q: What kind of protein should I take?
A: Plant-based protein is best, so go ahead and eat beans and legumes.

Q: Do people over the age of sixty-five lose muscle mass?
A: Yes, People over the age of sixty-five are more subject to losing muscle mass. By consuming more vegetables, one can reduce their risk of muscle mass reduction by half.

Q: What about an older person on bed rest?
A: Studies show that people over the age of sixty-five on bed rest lose muscle mass six times as much as younger people on bed rest.

Q: Why does this happen as we age?
A: As we age our kidneys start to decline and it may also be due to the acid-based diet that we tend to consume.

Q: Is muscle mass loss inevitable as we age?
A: No. Muscle mass loss with age is not inevitable. You just have to put in some effort. Adding protein does not seem to matter. A Japanese study showed that many elderly males actually increased their muscle mass, but they did put in the effort.

Q: What about younger people that eat a lot of protein?
A: People under the age of sixty-five who eat a lot of meat, eggs and dairy are seventy-three times as likely to die of diabetes. People in the moderate group were twenty-three times more likely to die of diabetes, compared to the base group which was consuming 50g of protein per day.[17]

Q: Can I live longer by consuming less protein?
A: Likely, yes! Studies show that a lower intake of protein consumption is shown to elongate life and eliminate or lessen the likelihood of disease in any age.

ASK DR. LIZ #27

PRUNES FOR OSTEOPOROSIS!

Q: How many people suffer from osteoporosis?
A: One in three older women will suffer from osteoporosis. Over 10 million Americans suffer from it. We are in an epidemic of osteoporosis.

Q: What can actually help protect against osteoporosis?
A: Evidence from a variety of studies show fruits and vegetables help protect bone health, such as bone mineral density. Bone health isn't just about calcium. Fruits and beans both are shown to reduce likelihood of hip fracture. Two different fruits that were tested included dried plums and dried apple rings. Both are shown to have bone protective effects. Prunes were more powerful than apples in protecting against bone loss and improving bone health.[18]

Q: What types of bone cells are involved?
A: Osteoblasts are bone-forming cells, and osteoclasts chisel away old bone. Too many free radicals may lead to excessive bone cell break down. It is found that oxidative stress helps cause osteoporosis. Fruits and vegetables help prevent against oxidative stress, which in turn helps to protect against osteoporosis, bone cessation, and bone formation.

Q. What about antioxidant rich fruits?
A. Yes. Antioxidant rich fruits help to prevent osteoporosis. Prunes, which are dehydrated plums, were actually tested and proven to help protect bone mineral density in the arm bone and the spine. This is true in both preventing and protecting bone mass. Hats off to strong bones!

ASK DR. LIZ #28

SEAWEED

Q: Are seaweed and kelp healthy for my body?
A: Yes. If you have ever had sushi, you've likely eaten seaweed wrapped around a sushi roll. If you've had miso soup, often there is seaweed in the soup, as well. You may also purchase seaweed sheets at the supermarket. Those make for a delicious salty snack! We know that vegetables are good for us, but you may not know that sea vegetables should also be included in a healthy diet. Seaweed and kelp are filled with phytonutrients and antioxidants, calcium, and a broad range of vitamins. Kelp is a type of brown seaweed found in oceans throughout the world. Seaweed is available in many varieties, including wakame and kombu, which are popular in Japanese cuisine, and dulse, which can be found on the coasts of Ireland and Maine. People with thyroid problems should consult their physician before consuming seaweed because it is high in iodine.

Q: What are the benefits of eating kelp and seaweed?
A: Seaweed is rich with nutrients, but that doesn't begin to scratch the surface of this fascinating food! Seaweed's best known benefit is it contains an extraordinary source of iodine, a nutrient missing in nearly every other food! Iodine is good for the thyroid, a gland in your neck. This helps produce and regulate hormones!

A malfunctioning thyroid can result in a wide range of symptoms such as fatigue, muscle weakness, and high cholesterol to name a few. In severe or untreated cases, it can lead to serious medical conditions like goiter (a swelling of the thyroid gland), heart palpitations, and impaired memory.

Seaweed can also regulate estrogen and estradiol levels, two hormones responsible for proper development and function of sexual organs. It can potentially reduce the risk of breast cancer. Seaweed also helps prevent inflammation, which can contribute to arthritis, celiac disease, asthma, depression, and obesity.

Q: Where can I purchase seaweed?
A: Take a trip to your local oriental market and get some seaweed. Any Thai restaurant should also serve seaweed as a side. Just ask for it!

ASK DR. LIZ #29

SESAME SEEDS

Q: Can you tell me about the health benefits of sesame seeds?
A: There are many health benefits that sesame seeds provide, including lowering cholesterol, lowering blood pressure, and decreasing inflammation enough so that it literally saves thousands of lives.

Q: Are there different types of sesame seeds?
A: There are white sesame seeds and black sesame seeds. Both are good and for different reasons.

Q: What is the difference?
A: Black sesame seeds contain 60 percent more calcium, contain higher levels of antioxidants, and in the Chinese culture, people consume black sesame seeds to protect their skin and hair from aging. Young women eat them to prevent anemia from menstruation.

Q: Is there anything specific about white sesame seeds that are beneficial that you can share?
A: The consumption of white sesame seeds has been shown to improve clinical signs and symptoms of osteoarthritic conditions of the knee. Ever since the 1920's, doctors have been injecting arthritis patients with gold. That's right, gold! Doctors are still using this disease-modifying anti-rheumatic drugs that are comprised of gold, which can slow the progression of rheumatoid arthritis. The problem is these drugs can be toxic.

Q: What does that have to do with white sesame seeds?
A: Injectable gold has been found to be beneficial, and has been in use for thousands of years. Researchers suspect that the sesame seed oil that is used as a carrier with the injectable gold drugs lowers inflammation.

Q: So, the sesame seeds are effective, not only the gold?
A: Yes! Recently there have been human studies on inflammation in people involving sesame seeds on osteoarthritis on inflammation.

Q: What did they find?
A: There have been measurable drops in inflammation in patients that have consumed white sesame seeds.

Q: What happened to their pain level?
A: Fifty patients were tested and put on sesame seeds for two months. On a scale of 1 of 10, each patient had a pain level at a 9 or 10. After consuming the white sesame seeds, their pain was reduced to a 3.5. Significant improvement in these patients with osteoarthritic conditions in their knee!

Q: How many sesame seeds did they need to consume?

A: Just one tablespoon per day of white sesame seeds! I am going to do my best to incorporate both white and black sesame seeds into my diet each day! I will sprinkle them on my cereal, eggs, mix them in smoothies, and put them in soups or over a steak!

ASK DR. LIZ #30

FOODS FOR BETTER SEX

Q: Can certain foods improve sexual experience?
A: Certain foods can effect sexual experience by improving blood flow while lessening inflammation in the pelvic region, both short term and long term. Interestingly, "heart" healthy changes are "sex" healthy changes! For example, high cholesterol may mean lower sexual arousal; therefore, by lowering cholesterol, you will be improving heart health, which may mean greater sexual arousal.

Q: What do we eat to improve sexual function?
A: Eat more vegetables, seeds, nuts, fruits, fiber, and beans. It is important to include in your diet high amounts of fiber and low amounts of saturated fats.

Q: Does this apply for both men and women?
A: Yes, it sure does!

Q: What does fiber have to do with sex?
A: Studies show that those who eat the most fiber are found to have the lowest amount of inflammation, as is measured in C-reactive protein. When there is less inflammation, often it is easier to become sexually aroused.

Q: What is Interleukin-18?
A: It is a protein which is a pro inflammatory cytokine, and it is a strong indicator of cardiovascular health.

Q: What foods would you recommend for a long life and love life for men?
A: A group of researchers put impotent men on a Mediterranean diet, 37 percent of the men regained normal sexual function. Similar benefits were found in women.

Q: What foods specifically improved erectile dysfunction?
A: Improvements in erectile function were tied to five things: increased intake of fruits, vegetables, nuts, beans, and a higher ratio of plant fats to animal fats.

Q. Is it true that high cholesterol impacts a woman's ability of sexual arousal?
A: Yes. It is believed to be detrimental due to the inflammation involved with high cholesterol. When consuming a plant-based diet, because of the anti-inflammatory and antioxidant benefits of a plant-based diet, a female's sexual function improves.

ASK DR. LIZ #31

QUIT SMOKING

Q: What is it about smoking that makes it so difficult to quit?
A: Smoking is typically an addiction, which makes it difficult to stop. Addiction of any sort is difficult to stop. Whether the habit of smoking involves nicotine, cannabis, or something else, it can be extremely difficult to quit.

Q: How does one go about stopping smoking?
A: Chinese medicine can be used effectively to help stop smoking; in fact, it can be used to treat any kind of an addiction. Often, an acupuncturist will use a combination of acupuncture, auricular therapy, and Chinese herbs to effectively treat addiction.

Q: How exactly does it work?
A: When a person is attached to something, be it smoking, alcohol, amphetamines, opioids, pornography, or something else, the neurotransmitters in the brain change. Multiple neurotransmitter systems reproduce themselves causing a more intense need for the substance. Treatment incorporates this into the strategy to ensure its effectiveness.

Q: How does the acupuncture, auricular therapy, and herbal remedy to effectively treat addiction?
A: Various points on the skin external to the ear can effectively send messages to the brain and help ease withdrawal symptoms and ease cravings by possibly reducing cortisol and balancing dopamine levels.

ASK DR. LIZ #32

TEA TIME

Q: What kind of healthy teas can keep you healthy and cool during the summer time?
A: Green tea, white tea, and licorice tea are three teas that are cooling or neutral in nature.

Q: What tea do you like to drink in the hot summer?
A: I really appreciate the benefits of green tea, especially in the summer time. Green tea clears heat and can help prevent heat stroke. It quenches thirst and promotes production of body fluids, so you are less likely to dehydrate in the hot sun.

Q: What benefits does white tea have?
A: White tea is also cooling in nature. It will also help keep you cool in the summer time. I like it because it is very light and refreshing.

Q: What about licorice tea?
A: Licorice tea is nice, as well. In fact, it is arguably a tea with many amazing benefits!
Licorice tea has anti-inflammatory properties that may ease the pain of arthritis. It also helps protect the stomach lining, can benefit bronchial disorders, and can help treat liver disorders such as hepatitis. Licorice can help prevent plaque in the vessels and help prevent heart disease; however, it should not be taken daily for more than three weeks as it can cause edema over time. You should check with your doctor to ensure it will not cause adverse reactions to any medications you are currently on.

Q: What are some more benefits of consuming green tea?
A: Green Tea is my favorite! It's loaded with antioxidants and helps improve brain function.
It helps to prevent Alzheimer's disease and has anti-anxiety effects. It also can boost your metabolic rate and lower your risk for cancer, including breast cancer, prostate cancer, and colorectal cancer. It can help lower your risk for type 2 diabetes.

ASK DR. LIZ #33

VITAMIN D: THE "SUNSHINE" VITAMIN

Q: What is vitamin D good for?
A: Vitamin D is so very good for many things. Clinical trials have shown vitamin D's preventative benefits range from cancer to high blood pressure to the swine flu, and fibromyalgia.

Q: Is it important to have enough vitamin D?
A: It sure is! Adequate intake of vitamin D is important for the regulation of calcium and phosphorus absorption. This proper balance provides us with healthy bones and teeth and is suggested to supply a protective effect against multiple diseases and conditions including heart disease, multiple sclerosis, type 1 and type 2 diabetes, including insulin resistance. Vitamin D was actually discovered by scientists in the early twentieth century when they were looking for a cure for rickets. Many studies have been conducted since, showing a powerful assistance to prevention for many diseases. The overall result is beneficial in reducing the risk of adverse health risks overall.

Q: Is vitamin D healthy for my skin?
A: Vitamin D contributes to skin cell growth, repair, and metabolism. It optimizes the skin's immune system and destroys free radicals that cause the body to age prematurely. Other vitamins that are good for your skin include vitamins A, B complex, C, E, and K.

Q: What kind of vitamin is vitamin D?
A: Vitamin D is a fat-soluble vitamin, as is vitamins A, E, and K.

Q: Can I get vitamin D from the sun?
A: Vitamin D can be absorbed through the skin and eyes. As we get older, our skin is less likely to absorb vitamin D as effectively. It's a good idea to get your vitamin D count checked when you go for your annual checkup with your doctor.

Q: How much vitamin D is healthy?
A: Most adults can benefit by taking 1,000 to 4,000 IU of vitamin D daily. The recommended for of vitamin D is vitamin D3, or cholecalciferol. Vitamin D2 is also okay.

Q: Can vitamin D help with fibromyalgia?
A: Yes! Vitamin D is known to help many fibromyalgia patients.

Q: Does vitamin D actually decrease pain?
A: Yes! Vitamin D has been shown to actually lower levels of pain in fibromyalgia patients!

Q: What if someone suffers from a vitamin D deficiency?
A: Not getting enough vitamin D can cause bone pain, muscle weakness, hypertension, and depression.

ASK DR. LIZ #34

WATERMELON

"Xi Gua"

Q: When I think of watermelon, I think of summertime, family, and fun! What do you think of when you think about watermelon?
A: Watermelon is a beautiful color pink, it's delicious, and it has many incredible health benefits!

Q: What are the health benefits of watermelon?
A: There are many! Watermelon is constitutionally cooling, making it a great idea to consume during the hot summer months! Whether you're out walking, golfing, swimming, or running errands, watermelon will keep you cool. In fact, watermelon is one of the very best "keep cool" foods on the planet! Watermelon can also help with wound healing, improve the immune system, reduce the risk of macular degeneration by helping to keep the retina healthy, and weight loss by reducing body fat!

Q: How does watermelon help reduce body fat?
A: The amino acid, citrulline helps to dissipate the accumulation of fat by converting it into Arginine, which in turn blocks the activity of TNAP (tissue non-specific alkaline phosphatase), which lessens the accumulation of fat cells in our body. Watermelon can also work as a natural Viagra.

Q: Watermelon can be used to treat erectile dysfunction?
A: Yes! This popular summer fruit dilates blood vessels much like Viagra and can potentially treat a mild ED without the side effects!

Q: Can watermelon do anything else?
A: Watermelon can also lower inflammation and be used to lessen conditions such as asthma, cancer, hepatitis, and provide sore muscle relief even better than ibuprofen! Watermelon actually works like a medicine. In fact, we are one of the few countries around the world that does NOT commonly use food as first line of treatment for disease.

Q: What is the history of watermelon?
A: Watermelon is believed to have originated in Africa in the Kalahari Desert, yet the Egyptians have cave paintings of men with watermelon over 5,000 years ago. The Chinese have used watermelon medicinally for thousands of years. Watermelon does grow in nearly one hundred countries around the world.

Q: What do they use watermelon for in the Far East?
A: In China, they call it Xi Gua! They use it for clearing "summer" heat and generating fluids. They use it to treat diabetes and hepatitis. It also helps to dry dampness that the body accumulates, and

dampness in the body can make us tired by causing fatigue and heaviness. Watermelon is also good for your heart, kidneys, and bone health!

Q: Is watermelon a fruit or a vegetable?
A: Some say watermelon is both a fruit and a vegetable. Others, interestingly say watermelon is NOT a fruit, but a vegetable! We do know that it's related to the cucumber, squash, and pumpkin. Either way, eat up! It's good for you!

ASK DR. LIZ #35

WEIGHT LOSS AND DIABETES

Q: Is it true that 2/3 of Americans are overweight?
A: Yes. By 2030, more than half our population may be clinically obese. Childhood obesity has tripled and most of them will grow up to be obese. The United States may be in the midst of raising the first generation since our nation's founding that will have a shorter predicted life span than that of the previous one.

Q: Does exercise play a role in weight loss?
A: Yes, but not enough. The food industry blames American obesity on inactivity, claiming Americans don't exercise enough. It may be true, but that does not explain or justify the number of overweight Americans. *"The increase of obesity can be explained by overconsumption of calories alone."* Exercise can prevent weight gain, but you would have to do a lot of it. Studies actually show that Americans have increased the amount of exercise they do, yet the number of overweight Americans has significantly increased.

Q: Why don't we lose more weight from exercise?
A: Part of it is that we don't get enough. A 1 percent decrease in BMI nationwide would prevent thousands of cases of diabetes. People tend to overestimate the number of calories that are burned from exercise.

Q: Does sexual activity cause weight loss?
A: Yes, but not enough. The average bout of sexual activity only lasts about six minutes, so a young man may burn twenty-one calories, which may burn one french fry worth of food intake.

Q: Is exercise good for us?
A: Absolutely! Getting your heart rate up is important to the health of your body. When we move, our blood moves, and it keeps what is known as our endothelium healthy. A healthy endothelium allows our body's own natural pharmacy to heal itself in most cases.

Q: So, it's important to exercise, but one must cut calories to lose weight?
A: Yes, studies show that obesity in the United States is primarily from consuming too many calories. In the 1980s, major food companies began to replace sugar with high fructose corn syrup. This is a problem because you eat and you don't get full, even though you are consuming many extra calories!

Q: What kind of food contains high fructose corn syrup?
A: Nearly everything contains high fructose corn syrup including tomato sauce, salad dressing, soda, many sports drinks, breads, breakfast cereals, ketchup, miracle whip, cough syrups, crackers, some yogurts, ice cream, cookies, cakes, and much more. You must read the food labels. Try to buy as many whole foods as you can. When you enter a grocery store, it's best to shop for most of your

foods on the perimeter of the store. Here, you will find whole food nutrition. Everything in the inside isles is processed.

Q: Are plant-based diets good for diabetes?
A: Yes. There is a 78 percent lower prevalence of diabetes when eating a plant-based diet. This is based on a study of 89,000 for over fifty years.

ASK DR. LIZ #36

FOODS FOR LONG LIFE

Q: Are there actually foods that will make us healthier and extend our life?
A: Yes. According to Taoists, there are indeed.

Q: Very interesting!
Can you tell us about some of these important foods for long life?
A: Black sesame seeds are one of the foods that are used for long life.

Q: What makes black sesame seeds so extraordinary?
A: Black sesame seeds are well known throughout Asia for their anti-aging properties. According to the Story of the Immortals, a woman named Lu could walk as fast as a deer and 300 li daily in her eighties. When asked for her secret to good health and vitality, she explained that she had been eating black sesame cakes all of her life! Black sesame seeds are really good for your blood. As we age, many of us, especially women, have less blood in our bodies. Black sesame seeds help to build our blood.

Q: What else do black sesame seeds do?
A: Black sesame seeds aid in digestion. They are good for the kidney and lung. Regular consumption of them will eliminate gray hair. It may take a couple of years but it works.

Q: How do you consume the sesame seeds?
A: I like to sprinkle a tablespoon on my cereal. yogurt, or in my smoothie daily.

Q: What is another food that the Taoist used for long life?
A: Peanuts! They were actually nicknamed "longevity nut." Peanuts are considered to be toxic and must be cooked raw.

Q: What is it that makes a peanut so special?
A: Peanuts have rich unsaturated fatty acids, vitamin E, and contain more than twenty kinds of nutrients and vitamins. Peanuts are wonderful for the brain!

Q: What about people who have an allergy to peanuts?
A: If you have a sensitivity or an allergy to peanuts, don't eat them. There are other wonderful foods that you can consume. Focus on those.

Q: Any good long-life food you can suggest for the holidays?
A: Chestnuts have many great qualities. Chestnuts were known as the king of the preserved fruits.

Q: What is it that make the chestnut so unique?
A: Chestnuts can strengthen the kidneys. They can also strengthen your tendons. This is really important because it can help prevent injuries. They are loaded with vitamins and fatty acids.

Q: Are they good for anyone with a particular disease?
A: According to Taoists, chestnuts are good for people with hypertension, coronary disease, and arteriosclerosis.

NOTES

1. Li Ling Lin, Ya-Hui Wang, et. Al, 2012. "Systems Biology of Meridians, Acupoints, and Chinese Herbs in Disease." https://www.ncbi.nlm.nih.gov/pmc/articles/PMC3483864/

2. Sook-Hyun Lee MS and Sabina Lim, KMD, PHD, 2017 "Clinical effectiveness of acupuncture on Parkinson disease". Ed. By Satyabrata Pany. https://www.ncbi.nlm.nih.gov/pmc/.articles/PMC5279085/.

3. Michael Greger, MD, May 22, 2013. "Breast Cancer Risk: Red Wine vs. White Wine." https://nutritionfacts.org/video/breast-cancer-risk-red-wine-vs-white-wine/

4. M. Beydoun, et al, July 9, 2020. "Large study links gum disease with dementia." https://nia.nih.gov/news/large-study-links-gum-disease-dementia

5. T.H.Chan, Harvard School of Public Health, 2012. "Impact of Fluoride on neurological development in children." https://hsph.harvard.edu/news/features/fluoride-childrens-health-grandjean-choi/.

6. Mehrdad Rafati Rahimzadeh, Mehravar Rafati Rahimzadeh, et al, Jan 11, 2022. https://www.bcbi.nlm.nih.gov/pmc/articles/PMC8767391/.

7. Harvard Health Publishing 2022. "Can you boost your memory by walking backward?" https://www.health.harvard.edu/mind-and-mood/can-you-boost-your-memory-by-walking-backward

8. Michael Greger, MD, FACLM, January 9, 2013. "Apple Skin: Peeling Back Cancer." https://nutritionfacts.org/video/apple-skin-peeling-back-cancer/
February 7, 2014

9. Michael Greger, MD, FACLM, May 10, 2013. "Which Fruit Fights Cancer Better?" https://www.nutritionfacts.org/video/.which-fruit-fights-cancer-better/

10. Hiya A. Mahmassani et al. 2018 "Avocado consumption and risk factors for heart disease: a systematic review and meta-analysis." https://www.pubmed.ncbi.nlm.nih.gov/.29635493/.

11. Michael Greger, MD, FACLM, Volume 17. "Foster Farms Responds to Chicken Salmonella Outbreaks." https://nutritionfacts.org/video/.foster-farms-responds-to-chicken-salmonella-outbreaks/.

12. Michael Greger, MD, FACLM, Volume 23, Mar 2015. "Do Antidepressant Drugs Really Work?" https://www.nutritionfacts.org/video/d0-antidepressant-drugs-really-work/

13. Michael Greger, MD, FACLM, Volume 25, Jun 2015. "What Causes Diabetes?" https://nutritionfacts.org/video/.what-causes-diabetes/.

14. Michael Greger, MD, FACLM, Aug 2015. "High Blood Pressure May Be a Choice" https://nutritionfacts.org/video/.hihg-blood-pressure-may-be-a-choie/.

15. Michael Greger, MD, FACLM. Mar 2015. "Nutritional Yeast to Prevent the Common Cold." https://www.nutritionalfacts.org/video/.nutritional-yeast-to-prevent-the-common-cold/.

16. Michael Greger, MD, FACLM. Jul 2014. "Which Nuts Fight Cancer Better?" http://www.nutritionfacts.org/video/.which-nuts-fight-cancer-better/.

17. Michael Greger, MD, FACLM. Jun 2016. "The Great Protein Fiasco" https://www.nutritionfacts.org/video/the-great-protein-fiasco/.

18. Michael Greger, MD, FACLM. Jul 2016. "Prunes for Osteoperosis" https://www.nutritionfacts.org/video/prunes-for-osteoperosis/.

REFERENCES

Beydoun M, et al, July 9, 2020. "Large study links gum disease with dementia."
https://nia.nih.gov/news/large-study-links-gum-disease-dementia

Chan T.H, Harvard School of Public Health,` 2012. "Impact of Fluoride on neurological development in children."
https://hsph.harvard.edu/news/features/fluoride-childrens-health-grandjean-choi/.

Cleveland Clinic. "6 Health Benefits of Corn." Nutrition. August 3, 2023.
https://health.clevelandclinic.org/.benefits-of-corn/amp/.

Flaws, Bob. "Chinese Medical Descriptions of Commonly Eaten Foods." In *The Tao of Healthy Eating*: Dietary Wisdom According to Chinese Medicine, 2nd ed. 62-97. Boulder: Blue Poppy Press, 2008.

Goldsmith, Ellen and Klein, Maya. *Nutritional Healing With Chinese Medicine*. Edited by Fina Scroppo. Toronto. Robert Rose Inc, 2017.

Greger, Michael. In *How Not to Die*: Discover the Foods Scientifically Proven to Prevent and Reverse Disease, 1st ed. New York. Flatiron Books, 2015.

Greger, Michael MD, FACLM, January 9, 2013. "Apple Skin: Peeling Back Cancer."
https://nutritionfacts.org/video/apple-skin-peeling-back-cancer/

Greger, Michael MD, FACLM, May 10, 2013. Which Fruit Fights Cancer Better?"
https://www.nutritionfacts.org/video/.which-fruit-fights-cancer-better/.

Greger, Michael MD, FACLM, Volume 17. "Foster Farms Responds to Chicken Salmonella Outbreaks."
https://nutritionfacts.org/video/.foster-farms-responds-to-chicken-salmonella-outbreaks/.

Greger, Michael MD, FACLM, Volume 23, Mar 2015. "Do Antidepressant Drugs ReallyWork?"
https://www.nutritionfacts.org/video/do-antidepressant-drugs-really-work/.

Greger, Michael MD, FACLM, Volume 25, Jun 2015. "What Causes Diabetes?"
https://nutritionfacts.org/video/.what-causes-diabetes/.

Greger, Michael MD, FACLM, Volume 29, March 2017. "Tea and Artery Function."
https://www.nutritionfacts.org/video/tea-and-artery-function/.

Greger, Michael MD, FACLM, Aug 2015. "High Blood Pressure May Be a Choice" https://nutritionfacts.org/video/.hihg-blood-pressure-may-be-a-choie/.

Greger, Michael MD, FACLM. Mar 2015. "Nutritional Yeast to Prevent the Common Cold." https://www.nutritionalfacts.org/video/.nutritional-yeast-to-prevent-the-common-cold/.

Greger, Michael MD, FACLM. Jul 2014. "Which Nuts Fight Cancer Better?" http://www.nutritionfacts.org/video/.which-nuts-fight-cancer-better/.

Greger, Michael MD, FACLM. Jun 2016. "The Great Protein Fiasco" https://www.nutritionfacts.org/video/the-great-protein-fiasco/.

Greger, Michael MD, FACLM. Jul 2016. "Prunes for Osteoperosis" https://www.nutritionfacts.org/video/prunes-for-osteoperosis/.

Gundry, Steven R. In *The Plant Paradox*: The Hidden Dangers In "Healthy" Foods That Cause Disease And Weight Gain, 1st ed. New York: Harper Collins Publishers, 2017.

Gundry, Steven R. In *The Plant Paradox Quick And Easy,* The 30-Day Plan to Lose Weight, Feel Great, and Live Lectin Free. New York: Harper Collins Publishers, 2019.

Harvard Health Publishing 2022. "Can you boost your memory by walking backward?" https://www.health.harvard.edu/mind-and-mood/can-you-boost-your-memory-by-walking-backward.

Jensen, Bernard. In *Foods That Heal*: A Guide To Understanding And Using The Healing Powers Of Natural Foods. Garden City Park, New York. Avery Publishing Group Inc. 1988.

Kastner, Jorg. In *Chinese Nutrition Therapy*: Dietetics in Traditional Chinese Medicine (TCM), 2nd ed. Stuttgart. Thieme, 2009

Kastner, Jorg. In *Chinese Nutrition Therapy*: Dietetics in Traditional Chinese Medicine (TCM)., 3rd ed. Stuttgart. Thieme, 2021.

Kendall, Donald E. In *Dao Of Chinese Medicine*: Understanding An Ancient Healing Art. New York. Oxford University Press, 2002.

Kim, H.B. In *Handbook of Oriental Medicine,* 5th ed. Acupuncture Media, 2015.

Koraneeyakijkulchai, Intra; Rianthong Phumsuay, Parunya Thiyajai, Siriporn Tuntipopipat, and Chawanphat Muangnoi. "Anti-Inflammatory Activity and Mechanism of Sweet Corn Extract on Il-lB-Induced Inflammation in a Human Retinal Pigment Epithelial Cell Line (ARPE-19)" Jan 27, 2023. https://www.ncbi.nlm.nih.gov/pmc/.articles/PMC9917234/

Lee, Sook-Hyun MS and Lim, Sabina KMD, PHD, 2017 "Clinical effectiveness of acupuncture on Parkinson disease". Ed. By Satyabrata Pany. https://www.ncbi.nlm.nih.gov/pmc/.articles/PMC5279085/.

Lin, Ling and wang, Ya-Hui, et. Al, 2012. "Systems Biology of Meridians, Acupoints, and Chinese Herbs in Disease." https://www.ncbi.nlm.nih.gov/pmc/articles/PMC3483864/

Mahmassani, Hiya A. et al. 2018 "Avocado consumption and risk factors for heart disease: a systematic review and meta-analysis." https://www.pubmed.ncbi.nlm.nih.gov/.29635493/.

Mohammad Azizur Rahman, Noorlidah Abdullah, and Norhaniza Aminudin. "Lentinula edodes (shiitake mushroom): An Assessment of in vitro anti-atherosclerotic bio-functionality." Saudi J. Biol Sci. accessed Feb 8, 2016. https://www.ncbi.nlm.nih.gov/pmc/.articles/PMC6302894/.

Nongdam P. and Leimapokpam Tikendra, "The Nutritional Facts of Bamboo Shoots and Their Usage as Important Traditional Foods of Northeast India." Hindawi. accessed July 20, 2014, https://www.ncbi.nlm.nih.gov/pmc/articles/PMC4897250/

Rahimzadeh, Mehrdad Rafati and Rahimzadeh, Mehrdad Rafati et al, Jan 11, 2022. https://www.bcbi.nlm.nih.gov/pmc/articles/PMC8767391/.

Rahman, Mohammad Azizur . Noorlidah Abdullah, and Norhaniza Aminudin. "Lentinula edodes (shiitake mushroom): An Assessment of in vitro anti-atherosclerotic bio-functionality." Saudi J. Biol Sci. accessed Feb 8, 2016. https://www.ncbi.nlm.nih.gov/pmc/.articles/PMC6302894/.

Rodrigues, Pedro. Tiago Ferreira, Elisabete Nascimento-Goncalves, Fernanda Seixas, Rui Miguel Gil da Costa, Tania Martins, Maria Joao Neuparth, Maria Joao Pires, Germano Lanzarin, Luis Felix, Carlos Venacio, Isabel C.F.R. Ferreira, Margarida M.S.M. Bastos, Rui Medeiros, Isabel Gaivao, Eduardo Rosa, and Paula A. Oliveira. "Dietary Supplementation with Chestnut (Castanea sativa) Reduces Abdominal Adiposity in FVB/n Mice: A Preliminary Study." Biomedicines MDPI. April 4, 2020. https://www.ncbi.nlm.nih.gov/pmc/.articles/PMC7235886/.

BIBLIOGRAPHY

Arooj M, Imran S, Inam-ur-Raheem M, Shahid Riaz Rajoka M, Sameen A, Siddique R, Sahar A, Tariq S, Riaz A, Hussain A, Sideeg A and Aadil RM. Food Sci Nutr. 2021 Jul
https://ncbi.nlm.nih.gov/pmc/.aeticles/PMC8269573

Arya SS, Salve AR and Chauhan S. J Food Sci Technol. 2016 Jan
https://www.ncbi.nlm.nih.gov/pmc/.articles/PMC4711439/.

Beydoun M., et al, July 9, 2020. "Large study links gum disease with dementia."
https://nia.nih.gov/news/large-study-links-gum-disease-dementia

Chan T.H, Harvard School of Public Health, 2012. "Impact of Fluoride on neurological development in children."
https://hsph.harvard.edu/news/features/fluoride-childrens-health-grandjean-choi/.

Cleveland Clinic. "Celery May Help Bring Your High Blood Pressure Down: Whole stalks provide more benefit than celery seeds." 2020, Dec 9.
https://health.clevelandclinic.org/celery-may-help-bring-your-high-blood-pressure-down/.

Cleveland Clinic. "6 Health Benefits of Corn." Nutrition. August 3, 2023.
https://health.clevelandclinic.org/.benefits-of-corn/amp/.

Couzin, Jennifer. "Volatile chemistry: children and antidepressants: more than a decade after doctors began prescribing SSRIs for young people, , investigators are trying to interpret ambiguous …". Science 305 (5683), 468-471, 2004

Flaws, Bob. "Chinese Medical Descriptions of Commonly Eaten Foods." In *The Tao of Healthy Eating*: Dietary Wisdom According to Chinese Medicine, 2nd ed. 62-97. Boulder: Blue Poppy Press, 2008.

Goldsmith, Ellen and Klein, Maya. *Nutritional Healing With Chinese Medicine*. Edited by Fina Scroppo. Toronto. Robert Rose Inc, 2017.

Greger, Michael. In *How Not to Die*: Discover the Foods Scientifically Proven to Prevent and Reverse Disease, 1st ed. New York. Flatiron Books, 2015.

Greger, Michael MD, FACLM, January 9, 2013. "Apple Skin: Peeling Back Cancer."
https://nutritionfacts.org/video/apple-skin-peeling-back-cancer/

Greger, Michael MD, FACLM, May 10, 2013. Which Fruit Fights Cancer Better?"
https://www.nutritionfacts.org/video/.which-fruit-fights-cancer-better/.

Greger, Michael MD, FACLM, Volume 17. "Foster Farms Responds to ChickenSalmonella Outbreaks."
https://nutritionfacts.org/video/.foster-farms-responds-to-chicken-salmonella-outbreaks/.

Greger, Michael MD, FACLM, Volume 23, Mar 2015. "Do Antidepressant Drugs ReallyWork?"
https://www.nutritionfacts.org/video/d0-antidepressant-drugs-really-work/

Greger, Michael MD, FACLM, Volume 29, March 2017. "Tea and Artery Function."
https://www.nutritionfacts.org/video/tea-and-artery-function/.

Greger, Michael MD, FACLM. Jul 2016. "Prunes for Osteoperosis"
https://www.nutritionfacts.org/video/prunes-for-osteoperosis/.

Gundry, Steven R. In *The Plant Paradox*: The Hidden Dangers In "Healthy" Foods That Cause Disease And Weight Gain, 1st ed. New York: Harper Collins Publishers, 2017.

Gundry, Steven R. In *The Plant Paradox Quick And Easy,* The 30-Day Plan to Lose Weight, Feel Great, and Live Lectin Free. New York: Harper Collins Publishers, 2019.

Harvard Health Publishing 2022. "Can you boost your memory by walking backward?"
https://www.health.harvard.edu/mind-and-mood/can-you-boost-your-memory-by-walking-backward

Health and Social Servics, *Nutritional Food Fact Sheet Series.*
https:www.hss.gov.nt.ca/en/.services/nutritional-food-fact-sheet-series/rabbit-and-hare#:~:text=Rabbit%20and%20hare%20meat%20are,active%20and%20to%20grow%20strong.

Jensen, Bernard. In *Foods That Heal*: A Guide To Understanding And Using The Healing Powers Of Natural Foods. Garden City Park, New York. Avery Publishing Group Inc. 1988.

Jingjing H, Hongna H, Xiaojiao W, Yan G, Yuexue Z, Yueqiang H. "Bie Jia Jian pill enhances the amelioration of bone mesenchymal stem cells on hepatocellular carcinoma progression." J Nat Med. 2022 Jan; 76(1):49-58 https://pubmed.ncbi.nlm.nih.gov/34297271/.

John Hopkins Medicine 2023. https://www.hopkinsmedicine.org/health/wellness-and-prevention/.ginger-benefits

Kastner, Jorg. In *Chinese Nutrition Therapy*: Dietetics in Traditional Chinese Medicine (TCM), 2nd ed. Stuttgart. Thieme, 2009

Kastner, Jorg. In *Chinese Nutrition Therapy*: Dietetics in Traditional Chinese Medicine (TCM)., 3rd ed. Stuttgart. Thieme, 2021.

Kendall, Donald E. In *Dao Of Chinese Medicine*: Understanding An Ancient Healing Art. New York. Oxford University Press, 2002.

Kim, H.B. In *Handbook of Oriental Medicine,* 5th ed. Acupuncture Media, 2015.

Koraneeyakijkulchai, Intrha; Phumsuay, Rianthong. Parunya Thiyajai, Siriporn Tuntipopipat, and Chawanphat Muangnoi. "Anti-Inflammatory Activity and Mechanism of Sweet Corn Extract on Il-1B-Induced Inflammation in a Human Retinal Pigment Epithelial Cell Line (ARPE-19)" Jan 27, 2023. https://www.ncbi.nlm.nih.gov/pmc/.articles/PMC9917234/.

Mahmassani, HA et al. 2018 "Avocado consumption and risk factors for heart disease: a systematic review and meta-analysis."
https://www.pubmed.ncbi.nlm.nih.gov/.29635493/.

Mayo Clinic Health System, 2021 May. "Radishes: Big flavor in a small package" https:www.mayoclinichealthsystem.org/.hometown-health/speaking-ofhealth/radishes-big-flavor-in-a-small-package.

Medicine (Baltimore). 2017 Jan; 96(3):e5836. "Clinical effectiveness of acupuncture on

Parkinson disease" ed. Satyabrata Pany. https://ncbi.nlm.nih.gov/pmc/.articles/PMC5279085/

Nongdam P. and Leimapokpam Tikendra, "The Nutritional Facts of Bamboo Shoots and Their Usage as Important Traditional Foods of Northeast India." Hindawi. accessed July 20, 2014, https://www.ncbi.nlm.nih.gov/pmc/articles/PMC4897250/

Rahman, Mohammad Azizur. Noorlidah Abdullah, and Norhaniza Aminudin. "Lentinula edodes (shiitake mushroom): An Assessment of in vitro anti-atherosclerotic bio-functionality." Saudi J. Biol Sci. accessed Feb 8, 2016. https://www.ncbi.nlm.nih.gov/pmc/.articles/PMC6302894/.

Rodrigues, Pedro. Tiago Ferreira, Elisabete Nascimento-Goncalves, Fernanda Seixas, Rui Miguel Gil da Costa, Tania Martins, Maria Joao Neuparth, Maria Joao Pires, Germano Lanzarin, Luis Felix, Carlos Venacio, Isabel C.F.R. Ferreira, Margarida M.S.M. Bastos, Rui Medeiros, Isabel Gaivao, Eduardo Rosa, and Paula A. Oliveira. "Dietary Supplementation with Chestnut (Castanea sativa) Reduces Abdominal Adiposity in FVB/n Mice: A Preliminary Study." Biomedicines MDPI. April 4, 2020. https://www.ncbi.nlm.nih.gov/pmc/.articles/PMC7235886/.

Saudi J. Biol Sci. 2018 Dec. https://ncbi.nlm.nih.gov/pmc/.articles?PMC6302894/.

University of Rochester Medical Center, "Kelp" 2023. https://www.urmc.rochester.edu/.encyclopedia/content.aspx?

UC Davis Health, "Potato health benefits and why you should eat more spuds" 2022 May. https://www.health.ucdavis.edu/blog/.good-food/potato-health-benefits-and-why-you-should-eat-more-spuds/2022/05

Xiao H, Deng Z, Hough JT, Chen X, Zhu Z, Lee J, Dominguez A, Shi T, Schmidt J, Bai Q, Wakefield MR, Fang Y. "The Effect of Asparagus Extract on Pancreatic Cancer: An Intriguing Surprise." Anticancer Res. 2022 May; 42(5):2425-2432. https://pubmed.ncbi.nih.gov/.355489758/